Cancer As A Wake-Up Call

An Oncologist's Integrative Approach To What You Can Do To Become Whole Again

M. Laura Nasi, MD

16pt

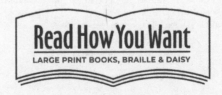

Read How You Want

LARGE PRINT BOOKS, BRAILLE & DAISY

Copyright Page from the Original Book

Published by
North Atlantic Books
Berkeley, California

Cover design by Howie Severson
Book design by Happenstance Type-O-Rama

Illustrations © 2018 by Paolina/Mariana Paolin (www.mundopaolina.com.ar)

Adapted from *El cáncer como camino de sanación*, translated from the Spanish by Estela Servente and edited by the author and Arnie Kotler.

Used by permission: From "Kindness" by Naomi Shihab Nye from *Words Under the Words: Selected Poems* by Naomi Shihab Nye, Copyright © 1995 by Naomi Shihab Nye. ˙

Printed in the United States of America

Cancer as a Wake-Up Call: An Oncologist's Integrative Approach to What You Can Do to Become Whole Again is sponsored and published by the Society for the Study of Native Arts and Sciences (dba North Atlantic Books), an educational nonprofit based in Berkeley, California, that collaborates with partners to develop cross-cultural perspectives, nurture holistic views of art, science, the humanities, and healing, and seed personal and global transformation by publishing work on the relationship of body, spirit, and nature.

North Atlantic Books' publications are available through most bookstores. For further information, visit our website at www.northatlanticbooks.com or call 800-733-3000.

Library of Congress Cataloging-in-Publication Data
Names: Nasi, M. Laura, author.
Title: Cancer as a wake-up call : an oncologist's integrative approach to
  what you can do to become whole again / M. Laura Nasi, MD.
Other titles: Cancer como camino de sanacion. Spanish
Description: Berkeley, California : North Atlantic Books, [2018] |
  Description based on print version record and CIP data provided by
  publisher; resource not viewed.
Identifiers: LCCN 2018007470 (print) | LCCN 2018024111 (ebook)

Subjects: LCSH: Cancer—Alternative treatment. | Cancer—Prevention. |
  Integrative medicine. | BISAC: HEALTH & FITNESS / Diseases / Cancer. |
  HEALTH & FITNESS / Alternative Therapies. | HEALTH & FITNESS / Diseases /
  General.
Classification: LCC RC271.A62 (ebook) | LCC RC271.A62 N3713 2018 (print) |
  DDC 616.99/4—dc23
LC record available at https://lccn.loc.gov/2018007470

1 2 3 4 5 6 7 8 9 KPC 22 21 20 19 18

Printed on recycled paper

North Atlantic Books is committed to the protection of our environment.
We partner with FSC-certified printers using soy-based inks
and print on recycled paper whenever possible.

TABLE OF CONTENTS

TABLE OF CONTENTS

PRAISE FOR CANCER AS A WAKE-UP CALL

"In *Cancer as a Wake-Up Call,* Dr. Nasi gifts us with an engaging and entertaining overview of holistic cancer care. This incredible resource presents a huge amount of information in easily digestible doses with the assistance of charming illustrations, valuable Take-Home Messages, and vital Practice for Healthy Living recommendations. The patient interactions and quotations from a host of international sages really help target the message. A must-read for anyone living with or beyond cancer, the people that love them, and hopefully, for their oncologists!"
—DONALD ABRAMS, MD, Chief of the Hematology-Oncology Division at San Francisco General Hospital, an integrative oncologist at the UCSF Osher Center for Integrative Medicine, Professor of Clinical Medicine at the University of California San Francisco, and editor (with Andrew Weil, MD) of *Integrative Oncology* (Oxford University Press).

"Dr. Laura Nasi is an internationally recognized figure in the field of integrative medicine. Her book, *Cancer as a Wake-Up Call* is intended for patients and family members dealing with cancer, and is a MUST-read for medical oncologists and health professionals. This book is a welcome addition to the library of anyone interested in a holistic approach to cancer care or just simply interested in living a better and healthier life."

—GARY K. SCHWARTZ, MD, Chief of Hematology and Oncology, Columbia University School of Medicine, New York

"In her integrative and systemic approach to cancer, oncologist Laura Nasi attends to the biological, cognitive, social, ecological, and spiritual dimensions of health and healing. Her advice on how to improve our quality of life in all these dimensions will inspire not only cancer patients but anyone desiring to live a healthier and more fulfilling life."

—FRITJOF CAPRA, PhD, physicist, systems theorist, and author of *The Tao of Physics* and other international bestselling books

"In *Cancer as a Wake-Up Call,* Dr. Laura Nasi guides the reader through the importance of using an integrative approach to cancer care. To have the best possible outcomes and thrive as a cancer survivor, you must focus on healing the body, mind, and spirit. *Cancer as a Wake-Up Call* provides valuable advice and is an evidence-based resource to help foster cancer recovery."
—LORENZO COHEN, PhD, Professor and Director, Integrative Medicine Program, MD Anderson Cancer Center, Houston, Texas

"This book is for anyone with cancer, anyone who works with those who have cancer, and for all of us who know someone who has cancer. It offers a treasury of approaches to living with and beyond cancer, bringing holistic perspectives into focus as a path on the journey of cancer."
—ROSHI JOAN HALIFAX, PhD, Upaya Zen Center, Santa Fe, New Mexico,

author of *Standing at the Edge: Finding Freedom Where Fear and Courage Meet*

*To Jazmín,
who initiated me
on this healing journey*

FOREWORD

"I'm so sorry, but you have cancer," is one of the hardest things I've ever had to say. As physicians, we pray right along with our patients that the biopsy will be benign, that we will be the bearer of good news and relief rather than the messenger of the words everyone understandably fears. Even though many cancers are curable, the words, "You have cancer," can understandably thrust someone into a terrifying "fight-or-flight" stress response faster than you can say, "Boo!"

Anyone who faces a cancer diagnosis will likely need to move through the inevitable cocktail of emotions—fear, anxiety, grief, insecurity, and sometimes shame, humiliation, or embarrassment. There's no bypassing these beautifully human emotions, which tend to get lit up when our very survival feels threatened. But what if it's possible to move through those emotions fully and quickly? What if on the other side of these contracted feelings lives an expansive curiosity? What if cancer is not necessarily a death sentence, but an opportunity for awakening, a portal to possibility? What if cancer is a wake-up call, inviting—even demanding—us to examine our lives and enter into a period of humble inquiry about where our lives might be out of alignment with our deepest truth?

Please feel my deep care when I say, with great sincerity, that I'm not suggesting that cancer is your fault. Even if you've knowingly engaged in behaviors that carry cancer risk, blaming or shaming yourself physiologically impedes the healing process, so the invitation is to let those emotions move through you like a wave, feel their pain, get help if you need to, and let them go. Cancer is an opportunity to hold a paradox. What if you're responsible *to* your illness but not *for* your illness?

Try getting curious instead. Enter into a state of wondering. Be willing to ask yourself, "If cancer is here as a wake-up call, what is its message for me?" Pay attention to the first answer that arises. In my work with tens of thousands of patients and thousands of physicians, you'd be shocked how often your first instinct is the most illuminating.

Notice next how you feel in response to what your intuition just told you. Maybe you asked your cancer, "What is your message for me?" and your cancer said, "You have to stop selling your soul at a job that asks you to violate your integrity" or "You've got to quit being a doormat in your marriage" or "You have to stop giving until you're depleted and prioritize your own needs." Maybe cancer said, "It's time to finally write that book you've always dreamed of writing!" or "You've just *got* to set boundaries with your abusive mother" or "Now is the time to twelve-step codependence" or "Baby, let's go on safari in Africa!"

Maybe your cancer is telling you to embark upon a spiritual retreat to reconnect with the Source of what enlivens you. Maybe cancer is here to help you quit smoking or to help you heal from childhood sexual abuse or get in touch with the fierce Mama Bear energy that can help you find your healthy *Rrrrrrrooooooaaaarrrr!* What if cancer is here to help you eat better, exercise more, and stop abusing toxic substances? What if cancer is here as a motivator to help you stop loathing your body and start treating it like a temple worthy of your devotion, care, and nourishment? What if cancer wants you to have more yummy sex and less toxic abuse from your boss?

In this illuminating book, Dr. Laura Nasi writes, "Cancer is a demand for change." For change to stick, change requires transformation. Cancer can be that transformational catalyst, if you let it. Dr. Nasi writes, "A disease might be the soul making its voice heard." If so, what is your soul saying? If you don't know, may this book help you discover what wants to awaken in you.

The fourteenth-century Sufi poet Jalaluddin Mevlana Rumi invites us into this kind of awakened alertness.

The breezes at dawn have secrets to tell you
Don't go back to sleep!
You must ask for what you really want.
Don't go back to sleep!
People are going back and forth

*Across the doorsill where the two
worlds touch,
The door is round and open
Don't go back to sleep!*

Oftentimes, cancer is a wake-up call, and then surgery or radiation or chemotherapy cures the cancer, and people go back to sleep. What if this is your opportunity to become and stay awake to the mysteries of life, the truth of your authentic nature, and the depth of your fully expressed Beingness? What if—*and I know this is a stretch*—cancer could even be a gift of love, an invitation to not just survive, but thrive? What if you are about to embark upon a hero's/heroine's journey that will change your life forever?

For four years, I created an art project called *The Woman Inside,* for which I cast the torsos of patients of mine who had breast cancer. I painted these sculptures with pigmented beeswax and then listened as these women told me their stories of the true nature yearning to break free from inside these plaster shells. As I listened to them tell their stories, I was shocked, as a young, naïve doctor, to hear so many of them say, "Cancer is the best thing that ever happened to me." How could that be? Was it possible? It seemed ludicrous, and yet some of these patients—the ones who didn't become contracted and embittered, the ones who found a portal out of their victim stories and took on the challenge cancer offered, the ones who said, "Hell yeah!" and dove into the dark places that had always frightened them—practically glowed with a brightness radiating from their shining eyes. Cancer had changed their life, and they were sincerely grateful. Some had not yet gone into remission, and the possibility of death still loomed, yet they were grateful even still.

I was in awe of these radiant women.

You could be next—if you're ready. Nobody can force your readiness, and if you're not yet ready to explore the dark shadows of your psyche and your life, be kind to yourself. Know that there is still hope for those with cancer who aren't yet ready for the deep soul work. It takes courage to dive into the unknown. But if there's even a spark of delicious excitement that arises, nourish yourself with this flicker. Dorothy Bernard said, "Courage is fear that has said its prayers."

May your fear say its prayers. May your journey be liberating. May this book be a blessing. May cancer be the best thing that ever happened to you.

With love,

Lissa Rankin, MD

New York Times best-selling author of *Mind Over Medicine, The Fear Cure,* and *The Anatomy of a Calling*

PREFACE

My Journey

I wrote *Cancer as a Wake-Up Call* to share what I've found most useful in my practice of Integrative Oncology. When I say *practice,* you might be picturing an office with a desk, chairs, an exam table, measuring devices, and so on. My practice is different. Since I began studying medicine more than thirty years ago, my ideas about consulting rooms and patients have changed.

I entered medical school at the University of Buenos Aires in 1984, the year following the return of democracy to Argentina. That year nearly 8,000 students entered medical school, twenty times more than had entered the year before. In these crowded conditions, my education was purely theoretical, with few opportunities for practical or hospital training. I graduated with honors, but that wasn't enough to secure a good residency. Entry at that time was by lottery rather than merit. But like the "good luck, bad luck" Chinese story, this encouraged me to continue my training in the United States.

Three years in an Internal Medicine Residency Program, followed by three years specializing in Clinical Oncology, were challenging personally and rewarding professionally. Memorial Sloan Kettering Cancer Center in New York is considered one of the two best facilities for cancer research and treatment in the world. Being admitted to Sloan Kettering's Clinical and Oncology Research Program, specializing in oncology, was a great honor.

I was one of the few Latin Americans admitted to the program, and under circumstances that felt like divine intervention. On the day of my interview, a historic blizzard struck New York, and two of my three interviewers weren't able to get to the hospital. The third, a lab scientist, asked only technical questions, while I've always focused on the human aspects of medicine. I left his office feeling discouraged. After the interview, I was invited to observe doctors at work, and I happened onto the office of Sloan

Kettering's Chief Medical Oncologist. It's an extremely busy practice, and the doctors there rarely stop, even for a moment, between patients.

When I walked in, I noticed that the Chief Doctor was taking a break for lunch, eating Chinese food his assistant had brought. So I introduced myself and told him I was disappointed I hadn't been interviewed by three doctors, like the other candidates. To my surprise, he grew engaged and asked about my interest in medicine, and specifically why I wanted to enter Sloan Kettering. Fifteen days later, I received a letter of admittance. I completed the specialization, gaining real knowledge about people suffering from cancer.

Following my fellowship, I was based in Switzerland for five years, working in the coordination center of the International Breast Cancer Study Group. This gave me the opportunity to audit and become familiar with hospitals throughout Europe, from Paris to Sarajevo, and also in Asia and Latin America.

After that, I worked for a Swiss pharmaceutical company, where I was in charge of a team that traveled around the world to find new molecules that might prove promising for developing anticancer treatments. We discovered a molecule in a Japanese lab that seemed like it might be the next blockbuster in oncology. After studying the molecule extensively followed by a week of due diligence in Tokyo, then submitting the results to our company's business team, no license agreement was reached, and the molecule remained "sitting on the shelf."

That disappointment was a milestone in my professional life. I realized that while I was spending time on a project that was dependent on economic factors, people were dying of cancer. I found that deeply unsettling, exacerbated by the realization that the paradigm I was immersed in viewed cancer very narrowly and was probably leading us the wrong way. Attempting to discover a cure for cancer only by looking through a microscope at the cells that are part of a tumor seemed myopic. We know there's a permanent dialogue between cancer cells and the immune system, so how could we suggest a treatment that doesn't take *the person* into account, the life challenges they're facing, and how their emotions might be affecting their well-being?

I found myself in a professional as well as a personal crisis. My husband at the time was a widower, and I'd raised his two beautiful daughters as my own. Still, I wanted to have a child. After undergoing fertility treatments for several years, I became pregnant with Jazmín, who then passed away before she was born. At that moment I realized that conventional medicine can play only a limited role in what we call health, and I needed to look at my whole life to discover what might help me get pregnant again.

Thanks to Jazmín, I embarked on a journey of personal integration. I took a yearlong sabbatical to contemplate what was important to me. I had a sense that if I visited people on the other side of the world whose bodies and biology were similar to mine but who had different beliefs and thought-structures, I might learn how our thoughts and beliefs mold us. I walked the Camino de Santiago pilgrimage route in Spain; then I headed to India for three magical months.

Elated by the birth of my first godson in Argentina, I returned to Buenos Aires and pondered how to integrate the spiritual worlds I'd been immersed in with my everyday life and scientific background. Returning to that special feeling of Argentine society, always fertile and creative—there's an energy that flows invisibly and unites us through good times and bad—drew me back in, and I decided to stay and to practice a different kind of medicine. During the next few months, I met with many health professionals who were also developing a more integrative approach to medicine and especially oncology. They referred to this approach as human, integral, integrative, and holistic and were determined to understand the health/disease process. All of us agreed that it's necessary to include more than just the body, but the person as a whole—mind, body, and spirit.

I became part of a group of healthcare professionals and therapists in Argentina who founded the Integrative Oncology Association to promote this perspective. I was invited to build, together with other professionals, the first integrative medicine team working at an academic institution in Buenos Aires, where hospital inpatients were treated with mind-body techniques such as relaxation and reflexology. Little by little, I began to develop new ways to treat people with cancer. I found that to begin to understand why a person got sick, I needed at least a two-hour first consultation. I'd explain that my intention was not only to take a snapshot of them, but also to view the video—the arc of their life with everything in it. I realized that if I gave enough time to listening, I could help the person see that they already knew what was making them sick. When I asked if they were living a more-or-less good life, almost everyone responded, in one way or another, "My life's a mess. I knew that if I kept up like this, I'd get sick."

We encountered a great deal of resistance from other medical sectors in Argentina, but I continued to incorporate mind-body techniques I'd learned in places including the Mind-Body Medicine Institute at Harvard, such as meditation, visualizations, and other spiritual techniques. I also brought in the advances we were learning from neuroscience and psycho-neuro-immuno-endocrinology. Thanks to discovering this widened perspective, I joined the group of pioneers, and together we've been developing a new paradigm for understanding cancer and the health/disease process. I firmly believe that healing requires looking at people as a whole, helping them become aware of the life they are living and addressing and modifying the things that are making them sick. It's not always easy to forge one's way against convention, but I can't see any other way to practice medicine effectively.

There are many ways to share this vision. One is trying to show other physicians the value of an integrative approach. Even more important, I feel, is to use this approach in my consultations and share the results with the general public, especially those who are suffering from cancer, and their families. I wrote this book to encourage readers to become familiar with integrative oncology and to take hold of the reins of their own journey to recovery.

The kick start for writing this book was given by Nora, a patient you'll meet in chapter 1, "The Diagnosis Is a Tsunami." "When I went to visit my oncologist," she told me, "I saw a small book that explains cancer and the effects of chemo and radiation. Why isn't there a book that tells you what you can do to feel better?" I hope this book will provide you with the tools you need to reclaim your life and your health, and encourage you to see cancer not as a final judgment but as a challenge to live a healthier, happier, more fulfilling life. And for readers who are at the end of life's journey, I hope this book helps you die in peace with a sense of completion.

—M. Laura Nasi, MD

April 2018

ACKNOWLEDGMENTS

If the only prayer you ever say in your entire life is thank you, it will be enough.

—MEISTER ECKHART

Thanks to my parents and my family of origin, who have always trusted me. Undoubtedly, this kind of support gives us the strength to continue our way. To my father, who taught me to face the most challenging interviews, saying, "Laura, remember that they have two legs and two arms just like you." To my mother, who gave me wings to fly. To my brothers, who initiated me into the worlds of exploring, playing, learning, sharing, crying, yelling, and smiling. And as the family continued growing, each lovely daughter of my heart, my sisters-in-law, my brother-in-law and my nephews, who bring a different tint into my life, allowing the picture to include the full range of colors. Thanks also to my companion in life, Fernando, who supports and encourages me to keep on exploring.

Thanks to life,[1] which has given me friends and colleagues to walk alongside, to everyone from whom I've received support, confidence, encouragement, and who at times, have helped me see my own shadow.

Thanks to my life for all who came and still come to my office seeking relief, caring, and the possibility of gaining a new perspective on what they're living with. Thanks to Nora, Silvia, Sebastián, Stella Maris, Martina, Mercedes, Zulma, Pilar, Estéfano, Irene, Isabelle, María Gabriela, Yanina, and to all who inspired me to write about the cases of this book. To each and all who teach me and allow me to unfold other parts of my being. Every encounter is a treasure. I feel privileged to be able to share intimate moments with individuals whose lives are flowering, and I feel honored to be able to accompany them along the way. Few professions can provide so much richness and satisfaction.

Thanks to my life for the masters I came to know and for those who guided me through their books: Carl Gustav Jung, Fritjof Capra, Anthony de Mello, Richard Moss, Yogi Bhajan, Carl Simonton, Amit Goswami, Deepak Chopra, Lawrence LeShan, Caroline Myss, James Oschman, Larry Dossey, Anselm Grün, Eugenio Carutti, Melanie Reinhart, Dane Rudhyar, Rupert Sheldrake, Bruce Lipton, Richard Gerber, Adriana Schnake, Stanislav Grof, Nassim Haramein, John Welwood, Keiron Le Grice, David Servan-Schreiber, Jeremy Geffen, Michael Singer, Susan Sontag, Ervin László, Ken Wilber, Eckhart Tolle, Carl Rogers, Ruediger Dahlke and Thorwald Dethlefsen, Candace Pert, Viktor Frankl, Tarthang Tulku, and many others whose seeds have germinated in me.

Thank you to my life for all those beings of light who have shown us the way: Gautama Buddha, Jesus, Mother Mary, Saint Francis of Assisi, Saint Teresa of Calcutta, and the many others who guide us in our days.

Thanks to Mariana Paolin for the heartful illustrations that make the text more accessible, to Naomi Shihab Nye for permission to quote from her beautiful poem "Kindness," and to Estela Servente and her team, who initiated the initial translations that made it possible for *Cancer as a Wake-Up Call* to be published in the US and beyond.

A very special thank-you to Arnie Kotler, whose editing, accompaniment through the publishing process, and advice have been invaluable. Thanks to North Atlantic Books for being open to a new and foreign writer. Since my first meetings with publisher Tim McKee and editors Pam Berkman and Louis Swaim, I've been happy working with a team committed to doing their work in a conscious manner, mindful of the impact they have on so many others.

Sincere thanks to Gary K. Schwartz, MD, whom I remember dearly as one of the best mentors I had at MSKCC; and to Donald Abrams, MD; Edward Bruera, MD; Lorenzo Cohen, PhD; Fritjof Capra, PhD; and Roshi Joan Halifax, PhD, for their kind and important endorsements.

A very special thanks to Dr. Lissa Rankin for writing the foreword to *Cancer as a Wake-Up Call.* When I first met Dr. Rankin at an Institute of Noetic

Sciences conference, I resonated with each word she expressed. I admire her courage in speaking out to reinforce this change in paradigm, and she does it in such an honest, scientifically sound, and loving way that I am sure her message is getting across to many people, and especially to health professionals who need to hear this from someone with her experience and authority. It was a surprise and an honor when she agreed to write the foreword to this book.

And finally, thanks to everyone who has shown interest in my book, encouraged me along the way, helping me realize my wish to share my experiences guiding cancer patients and their families.

INTRODUCTION

Do not believe in anything simply because you've heard it.

Do not believe in traditions simply because they've been handed down for generations.

Do not believe in anything simply because it's spoken and rumored by many....

Do not believe in anything merely on the authority of your teachers or elders.

But after observation and analysis, if you find that something agrees with reason and is conducive to the benefit of one and all, you can accept and live up to it.

—BUDDHA

Do not believe in anything simply because an external authority pronounces it. It won't be *your* truth until proven that it works for you. What *is* your truth?

Each of us is unique. Even when two people suffer the same kind of cancer, what led one to develop the disease might be very different from what led the other to develop it. This is why it's so important to look at each person, not just as a photo of a moment (e.g. a forty-one-year-old female with breast cancer), but to discover the film of her history and explore what led to this imbalance in her life.

Our life today is, in part, the result of decisions we made yesterday. In the same way, today's decisions shape our future. The physician's role is to help us identify possible stress factors that might have knocked us off balance and to help us reconnect with the neglected parts of ourselves, to find the thread that will lead us back to health.

Even today, in the twenty-first century, after so many years of cancer spreading throughout the populace nearly unchecked, we continue to cling to old hypotheses about cancer, causing millions of people to suffer and convincing them not to open up to new treatment possibilities. Conventional Western medicine looks pretty much exclusively at the physical body. Other medical approaches, such as Chinese, Ayurvedic, Vibrational, Energy, and

Quantum medicine, consider a person's full range of body, mind, and spirit. Integrative medicine today combines the best of conventional medicine with the wisdom of other modalities and with recent advances in quantum medicine, neuroscience, and psycho-neuro-im-muno-endocrinology.

When we face cancer, the fear that arises forces us to face death *and* can prompt us to embark on new dimensions of inquiry. Cancer not only engenders fear, but also can awaken us to a journey of integration, rediscovering ourselves as a living, emotional, social, and spiritual being, redirecting us back to health.

I wrote this book for those who want a broader approach, who wish to take the reins of their recovery process and do something more than (just) chemo. It is an invitation to use one's own cancer or that of a loved one as an opening to the possibility of a fuller life, of bringing more life to each new day. The stories in this book are true. They are offered as examples to transmit these basic principles, but all the names and specific information have been modified to preserve confidentiality.

Depending on the stage of cancer you or your loved one is undergoing, you may want to read this book in different ways, even skipping some chapters to return to them later.

As this book was conceived from the point of view of the integrative medicine, the tools described are based on scientific evidence, research studies, or medical explanations.

Each chapter includes breakout boxes titled "Practice for Healthy Living," intended to help you incorporate (literally, introduce into the body) the information in a practical and intuitive (and less logical) way. You'll also find text boxes with conceptual information, and other boxes that propose a space for reflection to promote opening to new possibilities.

The appendices at the end of the book answer frequently asked questions. Because a food revolution is underway, I've devoted an appendix to nutrition and included an explanation of the chakra system.

This book provides insights valid at the time of publication in 2018, but knowledge is a living entity. Not only do new advances in science appear every day, we're also updating our understanding of who we are. Look for updates at the book's website, https://cancerasawakeupcallbook.com. I also welcome comments and questions emailed to cancerasawakeupcall@gmail.com.

I hope you will find in this book answers to your questions and doubts, and an invitation to understand the health/disease process as part of a journey you can take to increased self-knowledge and growth, recognizing that you are the principal actor of your treatment and recovery.

Medical Disclaimer

The contents of this book are for information purposes only and are not a substitute for professional medical advice, diagnosis, or treatment. Always seek the advice of your physician or other qualified healthcare provider with any questions you have regarding a medical condition and before undertaking any diet, dietary supplement, exercise, or other health program. Any application of the material set forth in the following pages is at the reader's discretion and is his or her sole responsibility. Neither the author nor the publisher is responsible for any adverse effects resulting from your use or reliance on any information contained in this book.

Chapter 1

THE DIAGNOSIS IS A TSUNAMI

The old man cries
Sorrow on people's faces
The tsunami

—PHEKO MOTAUNG

Nora, an administrative assistant at a textile manufacturing office, had been living with ovarian cancer for fifteen years when I met her. She'd had multiple recurrences, undergone surgeries, and was once again having chemotherapy. She was determined to have a different experience this time and wanted to know how that might be possible.

She told me the horror story of her diagnosis. After surgery to remove a cyst from her ovaries, the physician, a handsome young man she barely knew, told her, "Nora, we were surprised to find something behind the cyst. You *have advanced ovarian cancer." The words exploded in her head, and her whole body began to shake. It felt as though time had stopped, and she was unable to hear another word. "I saw him moving his lips, but I couldn't hear anything. It was a rainy Friday, July 24. I was thirty-nine-years old."*

A cancer diagnosis is one of the most traumatic experiences a person can have. Doomsday fears are stirred, and we might even go into shock. We regress to the mind of a helpless infant as the news punctures our world as we know it, removing all feelings of safety or refuge. Everything we take for granted is suddenly taken from us. Feelings so painful we can't even let them arise, threaten our ability to understand what's happening. The mind blurs; we lose lucidity and grounding. We're inconsolable; *everything* feels impossible.

This is the *emotional* reaction of the psyche, and the same is going on at the level of the body. Faced with danger, the body's alarm system, which is in the primitive part of the brain called the limbic system, activates. This fight, flight, or freeze reflex works on behalf of survival, while our neocortex, the newest and most developed part of the brain that's responsible for understanding logic, concepts, and complexity, short-circuits. Suddenly we're overtaken by fear, despair, and turmoil on the physical, emotional, social, and existential levels.

The limbic system coordinates emotions and behavior, integrating internal and external data, and activates changes in breathing, blood pressure, and other bodily functions through an instantaneous interaction with the endocrine system and the autonomic nervous system, which affects the entire *PNIE (psycho-neuro-immuno-endocrine) network.* (See box entitled "PNIE Network" for a description of the PNIE.) The amygdala, a basic structure of the limbic system, controls and mediates relevant emotions such as affection, aggression, and fear. When it's activated, we are on full alert. The amygdala is also involved in anxiety and emotional memory disorders.[1]

A cancer diagnosis is like a tsunami that propels us across the beach, threatening to drown us and destroy all the places we feel secure, including the seat of our identity. All known reference points are lost. In this climate of extreme urgency, all we want is to get out of the situation. In this state, it's next to impossible to make important treatment decisions. A cancer diagnosis falls like a stone hurled into the water, and its impact expands in concentric waves, reaching all family members, friends, colleagues, and even healthcare workers.

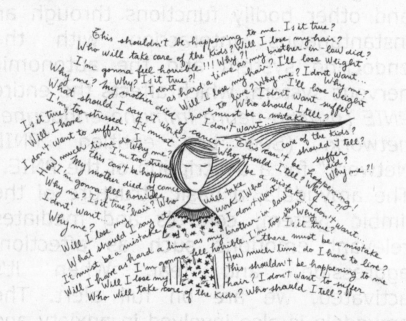

The diagnosis is a tsunami.

Recognizing that our health is more than just physical is not a new discovery, even in the Western allopathic setting. In 1948, the World Health Organization (WHO) defined health as "a state of complete physical, mental and social well-being and not merely the absence of disease or infirmity."[2] I would expand WHO's definition to add **spiritual well-being. Disease is a message from the soul. Attempting to restore health by attending only to its physical aspects is too limiting.**[3]

Whatever triggered the disease, **cancer invites us to stop,** to step out of the turmoil in which we are moving like a rat on a grid, to **find a new order.** It invites us to evaluate how we've been living, what we're not attending, and how we reached the point of disease; and then to ask ourselves, how might we be able to return to a healthy life? What is the soul trying to tell us? What makes us happiest? What is our right path?

Nora believed that cancer was an enemy that had come from the outside to attack her and that chemotherapy was the only solution. We talked for two hours, and I encouraged her to see cancer as a protest, rather than an enemy. A group of cells belonging to her own body had risen up and organized a strike, then a riot, indicating a system that was coming apart.

If cancer is an enemy, the only tactic is removing it, never recognizing that *cancer is a part of us* that needs attention. If we view cancer as an expression of imbalance, that something isn't working properly, a systemic uprising, we can study its message using an integrative overview. What is making those cells rise up? When we address the underlying issue, it's likely the manifestation will not recur.

Allopathic medicine sees the body as a machine, and either the part that isn't working is removed through surgery and replaced by another one, or the body is given medicine to repair the broken part or at minimum, to suppress the symptoms. But *we are more than machines.* I prefer the image of an organic garden. When a weed grows, we pull it out. But if that's all we do, another weed will grow back. **We need to improve the soil, to nourish the body, mind, and spirit with new approaches and lifestyle changes, addressing our whole self. This integral perspective, focusing on the person and not just the cancer, gives us a broader view of treatment. Cancer must be addressed directly and thoroughly, but how can we treat the ground so the weeds won't grow back?**

There are many factors behind the development of a disease. When several conspire, at a certain threshold we become sick. This helps explain why in a family that has a genetic mutation that indicates a likelihood for certain illnesses, only some family members get sick. We know cigarettes cause cancer,[4] but not all smokers contract it. For cancer to develop, several factors tend to be present: unhealthy lifestyle and dietary choices, inadequate exercise, and much more. Throughout our lives, more than once, we are all probably developing small cancers and our immune systems are controlling them or making them disappear.[5],[6]

Stress affects some people's hearts, while others under stress remain symptom-free. **Chronic stress challenges the immune system and makes us vulnerable to diseases,** including cancer. A combination of internal (e.g., anxiety) and external (e.g. divorce, death of a loved one, a hostile workplace) is responsible for making us more vulnerable to sickness, cofactors leading to a breakdown of the immune system.

An external factor that stresses one person may not affect another. Although many people get sick following a divorce, we can't say that divorces cause cancer. If that were the case, everyone who gets divorced would get cancer. But the fact that someone gets cancer in the midst of a stressful situation at minimum calls us to notice how we are living and encourages us to seek other ways of coping.

Medicine is not math, and the health/disease process is not an equation, but through the progress of science, we continue to connect factors not previously recognized as associated. This offers us clues; we understand that

the way we're living and the way we view the world can lead us to decisions and choices that make us sick.

The number of cancer diagnoses is increasing steadily. Although death from some types of cancer, such as leukemia and breast, prostate, and ovarian, is decreasing, incidence (new cases per year) is increasing.[7] And the number of new cases is expected to rise by as much as 70 percent over the next two decades.[8] **In the US, one in two men (half!) and one in three women (a third!) will develop cancer during their lifetime.**[9]

Wherever we live in the world, our twenty-first-century lifestyles are becoming Westernized, including diets low in nutrients and high in additives, sleep deprivation, sedentariness, high stress, relationships that don't address conflict, domestic violence, and isolation.

Is it True that the Number of Cancer Cases Is Rising Every Day?

Or is it because more cancers are detected earlier?

Screening is now so precise that it can detect small cancers that previously might not have been noticed during a person's lifetime. Although it's true that the number rises because cases previously undetected are now being diagnosed, statistics show that some types of cancer, e.g., lung cancer and melanoma, are increasing in some places in the world.[10]

This is quite different from the way our grandparents lived, without junk food or sugary drinks; when food was homemade; when children walked or rode bikes to school, played on the streets, and didn't have to face the insecurity, traffic, and social violence we know today. We lived in larger families offering a network of social support, with sleep cycles closer to the setting and rising of the sun. There was less pressure, less stimulation (cell phones, computers, electronic games, and so forth), and more outlets for creativity.

Among those in the US who don't smoke, the highest causal factors for getting cancer are an unhealthy diet and sedentariness. **Up to 60 percent of cancer cases could be avoided with a healthy diet, regular exercise, stress management, and refraining from smoking.** Some time ago we began to suspect that our current lifestyle could sicken us; now we are certain.

Veronica came to see me after she'd been diagnosed with breast cancer. She had been a yoga teacher and a vegetarian for many years, visiting ashrams in India frequently. She devoted her time to serving others. Now she felt hopeless. "Why me?" she asked. "I've been doing everything right. I eat properly, exercise, meditate, take care of my family, help the poor." Veronica's case required a deeper (or perhaps a wider) look.

Forty percent of new cancer diagnoses cannot be attributed to unhealthy diets, smoking, or sedentariness. Other possible factors include internal conflict, self-criticism and negative self-judgment, emotional instability, and existential dissatisfaction. We can't explain all cases in one way.

Understanding cancer not as an enemy, but as the manifestation of an imbalance, unhealthy habits, an unexpressed purpose of life, or the call of the soul requesting we find our true course empowers us to be on our own side and do what is needed for our benefit. Beyond medical treatment, we can **live a healthier and more balanced life, taking more responsibility for our own well-being.**

After surgery, Veronica experienced a recurrence of cancer and became so depressed, she lost her will to live. It took her weeks to accept that her cancer had come to stay, at least for a while. "Why have the tenants come back again?" she asked, referring to her tumors. "I want it to be different!" This protest represented Veronica's first steps toward flourishing, although she wasn't aware of it yet.

Veronica was ready to embark on a journey, not the trip to Europe she'd wanted for so long, but a tour back to herself. It would be a journey full of adventure and a profound satisfaction she could never have planned. Along the way, she learned to put the disease and the treatment in the right places in her psyche and began to focus on what would really give her the will to live.

She got a two-month leave from work to take the time and space she needed to embark on this journey to self-knowledge. We worked on some meditations and visualizations that led her to her family and ancestors. Based on these images arising in her, I suggested she study her family's genealogy. Through talks with her mother and her aunts recalling occurrences in the past, she began to meet family members throughout the world via Skype and email and connected to something larger than herself. "I've begun to understand where I come from, who I am," she told me with an air of confidence I hadn't seen before. Her extended family was becoming a part of her, something she had until then denied.

She returned to work on a part-time basis. Work issues were no longer consuming so much of her energy, and she became wildly enthusiastic about a family reunion project she was orchestrating on Facebook. I'd never seen her so happy.

Take-Home Message

Cancer invites us to stop and find a new order.

Paying attention only to physical symptoms is limited. Removing the weed (the tumor) is important, but it is equally important is to take care of the soil, the ground.

Let us accept that health is physical, mental, emotional, social, and spiritual well-being.

The way we live and the way we think can make us sick. Chronic stress and a lack of spiritual connection can make us vulnerable to disease.

One in two men and one in three women will develop cancer during their lifetimes.

Sixty percent of cancer cases can be avoided.

We can move to a healthy lifestyle that can bring our happiness back.

Chapter 2

SO ... WHAT IS CANCER?

How could they see anything but the shadows if they were never allowed to move their heads.
—PLATO, *THE ALLEGORY OF THE CAVE*

Cardiovascular diseases claim more lives than all forms of cancer combined, and **half of those diagnosed with cancer in First-World countries are cured.** Yet we are petrified of cancer.

Success Rates of Conventional Medicine

Fifty percent of those diagnosed with cancer are successfully cured by surgery, radiation, and chemotherapy. For some types of cancer, this number reaches 90 percent. When diagnosed early, many kinds of cancer can be cured with surgery. For other types of cancer, chemotherapy's curative efficacy goes far beyond the adversity it brings about. For example, chemo plays a key role in *curing* some leukemias, lymphomas, and testicular cancers.

Other chronic diseases can cause pain comparable to cancer, such as difficulty breathing after heart failure, learning to walk after a stroke, or undergoing dialysis to remove toxins when you have kidney disease. But none of these diseases induce as much fear as *cancer.* No other disease conjures such images of devastation and loneliness, and none threaten our self-image to so great an extent. Having cancer impacts our body, identity, sense of safety, and lifestyle. We feel devastated, completely undone.

In our collective view, cancer is inevitably linked to suffering, weight and hair loss, shortness of breath, loss of independence, and imminent death. This is not always the case. These things can happen during the disease's advanced stages, but not everyone diagnosed with cancer walks this path.

Pain and other adverse effects of cancer therapies such as nausea receive much better treatment today. Millions of people all over the world receive chemo and continue their normal lives, even going to work. People we pass on the street or those having coffee next to us at Starbucks might have just completed a cancer treatment, and we won't even notice. What we *think* about cancer can make us suffer more than what's actually going on.

The fear and tragedy we associate with cancer are, in part, what brings about our suffering. Many people find it difficult even to utter the word.

Updating the meaning of *cancer* can help us understand the actual condition and face each new day in the best possible way.

Carolina, a psychologist friend of mine, telephoned, filled with anxiety because she'd detected a lump in her breast and was about to have a biopsy. "Laura, is this procedure necessary?" she asked.

I told her it's not unusual to find suspicious lesions and normally they're benign. If it is malignant, it's much better to detect it early and receive good treatment. If there is any doubt, a biopsy is recommended to determine the nature of the lump and whether surgery is needed. The earlier the diagnosis and treatment, the greater the possibility of a cure.

Not that many years ago, the majority of those diagnosed with cancer lived just a short time. Today the number who live with and beyond cancer is increasing. This is especially true with children and with adults whose cancer is detected before it metastasizes.

The Word Cancer

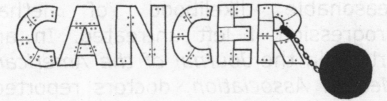

The heaviness of the word cancer.

The word *cancer* has such negative associations that some medical professionals are considering reserving it for the most severe cases.

Because of the heaviness of the word *cancer:*

• Some US oncologists are beginning to find other names for malignant tumors in order to prevent overtreatment.

• Doctors in Spain are attempting to reduce its stigmatization.

What sounds more severe: leukemia, lymphoma, or cancer? Neoplasm? Hyperplasia? Lesion or cell proliferation? Sarcoma, tumor, melanoma? Malignant polyp? Words are valanced by the devil. A group of physicians at the US National Cancer Institute has begun to consider whether the term *cancer* should be reserved for lesions that have a reasonable likelihood of lethal progression if left untreated. In an article in the *Journal of the American Medical Association,* doctors reported on the overdiagnosis and overtreatment of breast, lung, prostate, and thyroid cancers brought about by fear of the word *cancer.*[1]

"Although I understand everything you're telling me and at times I feel calm, mostly I'm really afraid. This feels stronger than I am. Why haven't we found a cure yet?"

I told Carolina cancer is not a single disease.

"Really? Then *what is cancer?*"

So ... *what is cancer?* Carolina's question echoed inside me in a slowly increasing crescendo, like the movement in Ravel's *Bolero,* and I wanted to find a comprehensive way of explaining the complexity of cancer.

The word *cancer* embraces hundreds of different diseases. Something similar happened with the word *infection* ninety years ago, before antibiotics. People with flu, plague, meningitis, or pneumonia had little chance of survival. Today we know that although they're all infections, each is a different disease with different treatments and prognoses.

Breast cancer is different from skin cancer, and not all breast cancers behave in the same way. Different cancer types and subtypes develop in unique ways and have entirely different prognoses. Some subtypes of lung cancer grow slowly, while others spread quickly. Some respond well to therapy, while others are difficult to treat.

When Cancer Spreads, Does It Keep the Same Name?

Cancer is always named after the part of the body where it starts. A breast cancer that spreads to the liver is called metastatic breast cancer and not liver cancer. Prostate cancer that spreads to the bones is referred to as prostate cancer that has metastasized to the bones.

In addition, each case is unique, just as each individual is unique. Two people may develop cancer in the same part of the body, but the disease's progression might vary depending on the response to therapy and the way each person lives the experience.

We call them all cancer, but actually they're a lot of different diseases. So, then, *what is cancer?* Carolina's question continued to echo within me.

Let's begin by looking at the **cell model,** which is widely used to explain and treat cancer. Our body is composed of 37.2 trillion living cells.[2] Normal cells grow, divide into new cells, and die in an orderly fashion. They cease to thrive when they come into contact with a neighboring cell. This is known as *contact inhibition.* Healthy cells observe the dictum, **"Your rights end where another's begin."**

A Brief History

Cancer is cited in ancient documents, among them Egyptian papyrus scrolls from around 1600BC. It's said that Hippocrates was the first person to use the term *karkinos* (a mythical giant crab). He noticed a tumor surrounded by veins on a person's neck and likened it to the body and the feet of a crab.

In 1858, a German physician named Rudolf Virchow observed that the disease started at a primary cell and then spread. Cancer was then a tumor, similar to a cauliflower, he said, resulting from a cell that mutated, became malignant, and started to grow in an uncontrolled manner. Extensive surgical and radiotherapeutic techniques were designed to remove and eradicate the disease, based on Virchow's cell theory.

During the twentieth century, in an atmosphere of world wars, cancer was likened to an enemy that invades other parts of the body and has to be vanquished.

During World War II, health workers observed that soldiers who'd been exposed to toxic gases developed low white blood cell counts. This led to the experimental use of toxic substances like mustard gas and its derivatives (mustines) to treat lymphomas. *Chemotherapeutic bombs* were developed that attacked cancer cells, and normal cells as well, leading to now well-known adverse effects. This was the birth of chemotherapy.

In 1971, Richard Nixon declared a war on cancer and supported new research initiatives with the intention of eradicating cancer as a primary cause of death.

Cancer begins when cells in some part of the body begin to grow in an unchecked manner and, instead of dying, proliferate in an out-of-control fashion. Mutated cells accumulate, form a tumor, and then invade other tissues or organs—either locally or at a distance. Cancer cells get into the bloodstream or the lymph vessels and travel to other parts of the body, where they grow and form new tumors. This cancer-spreading process is called *metastasis*. The uncontrolled growth patterns and the ways in which cancer cells invade other tissues determine whether they are malignant. According to this biological model, the problem is one of **proliferation and cell behavior disorders.**

Why do cancer cells undergo uncontrolled growth? Deoxyribonucleic acid (DNA)[3] is in the nucleus of every cell and carries in it instructions for the growth, development, functioning, and reproduction of every known living organism. An alteration in DNA, known as a genetic mutation, affects a gene's expression.

What Causes Mutations?

Mutations can be inherited or caused by carcinogens.

A person may have a **hereditary predisposition** to develop cancer if he or she is born with a genetic mutation, or a gene vulnerable to mutations. Only 5 to 10 percent of cancers are inherited. What is inherited is not the cancer but the gene that has a mutation which indicates an increased likelihood of developing cancer.

Mutations also occur as the result of **carcinogenic factors** such as cigarette smoke; pollution; asbestos; certain viruses, e.g., human papillomavirus (HPV) or Hepatitis B; exposure to UV radiation; and chemical products such as bisphenol A (BPA), commonly used to make plastics.

When a normal cell's DNA is altered, the cell either repairs itself or activates a mechanism known as programmed cell death to prevent the mutation from being passed to future generations. But in cancer cells, the damaged DNA is not repaired, and the mutated cell doesn't die. Instead, it multiplies uncontrollably, passing the mutation on to its daughter cells. This is a summary of the cell model of cancer.

Other researchers see cancer as a genetic disease. *So we must continue our inquiry ... what then is cancer?*

For about fifty years, we thought nearly all our health and destiny were preprogrammed in our genes. This is called genetic determinism, and it considered cancer to be the result of gene mutations and encouraged research in gene therapy, with the hope of delivering functional genes into a person's genome to replace genes with mutations.

Is a Mutated Gene Necessarily Cancer?

Mutated cells, whether inherited or altered by a carcinogen, don't necessarily develop into malignant cells. Being born with a genetic predisposition to the development of a certain type of cancer does not mean you will necessarily get cancer.

Recent findings in cellular biology show that our genetic *expression* is controlled by both internal and external environments. The experiences we undergo and the way we perceive affect our cells. Epigenetics studies how our interactions with the environment and the interactions of our recent ancestors affect genes, switching them on or off.[4]

Unhealthy stressors,[5] such as poor nutrition, hormonal imbalances, toxins and pollutants, chronic tension, and unresolved conflicts, can increase the likelihood that genes that might cause cancer will express. **Positive lifestyle choices, on the other hand, reduce the risks of developing cancer considerably and aid us in recovering our health.**

The Human Genome Project, completed in 2003, had the intention of identifying and mapping all the genes of the human genome, which is the complete set of nucleic acid sequence for *humans,* encoded as DNA. They did this so we might be able to identify the genetic alteration(s) corresponding to every disease and eradicate the mutated genes we inherit from our parents. Today, however, we know that **those with a hereditary predisposition to develop cancer represent a minority** and the effort to develop gene therapy has slowed down considerably.

By the time a cell becomes cancerous, it has already undergone multiple genetic alterations, affecting cell division. Mutations may have affected the genes that promote (oncogenes) or inhibit (tumorsuppressor genes) cell division. A mutated oncogene can promote cells to divide unhindered, like having your foot stuck on the gas pedal. A mutated tumor suppressor gene will not function properly suppressing tumors but will allow cells to reproduce unchecked, like a car with faulty brakes. This is the perspective of those who view cancer through the lens of genetic determinism.

Recent studies in molecular biology support the field cancerization model of carcinogenesis. First, a cell acquires a mutation and forms a *patch* of mutated daughter cells. This does not happen in isolated cells but in a *field* of mutated cells that were exposed to the same carcinogen. These cells continue to mutate, and since they're growing more rapidly than normal cells, they begin to replace them. When there is a field of cancerization, therapeutic procedures such as surgery or radiation need to treat more than just the tumor, but the whole affected field. Otherwise, if the adverse conditions continue,[6] it could lead to new tumors.

There are other perspectives on the question of why cancer cells or fields of cancer cells accumulate so many mutations and behave without control. So we must continue our inquiry ... *what is cancer?*

Some researchers explain these multiple mutations as a consequence of rapid cell division. The cells don't have time to repair mistakes before accumulating further mutations.[7] Other researchers state that, in the same way that bacteria attempt to adapt to a different media, cancer develops an accelerated mutation to generate more evolved cells.[8] And others explain the accelerated mutation as the result of the strong metabolic disorder in cancer cells. They view cancer as a metabolic disease.

The **metabolic model** is the result of twentieth-century research that received two Nobel prizes, both focusing on **alterations of the metabolic process in cancer cells.** The German physician Otto Warburg stated that cancer is produced by damage to normal cells' metabolism (oxidative or aerobic[9]), which brings about a lower rate of energy production (anaerobic metabolism). The damage, Warburg posited, can be induced by chemicals in processed food, some medications, and environmental pollution.[10] The resulting metabolic disorder creates instability in the cells that leads to genetic mutations that eventually produce cancer cells.

Since then, many treatments have been proposed based on nutrition and a chemical-free diet, vitamin and mineral supplements, and other substances that provide the cells with the oxygen needed to remove toxins. Later research challenged this theory by showing that energy-producing/sugar-breaking mechanisms in the cells are similar in both cancer and normal cells.[11] Although Warburg's hypothesis has never been proven, it has led to beneficial research on the effects of healthy food and supplements for the prevention and treatment of cancer.

The second Nobel Prize was awarded to Linus Pauling, who observed that high doses of vitamin C have beneficial effects on cancer patients. Based on this, high-dose vitamin and mineral therapies, known as orthomolecular medicine, have been proposed. Pauling's hypothesis on the positive effects of vitamin C on cancer patients has also not been proven.[12] Nonetheless, based on Pauling's preliminary findings, many support this kind of therapy.

The above models focus on the body, treating the human being, more or less, as a sack of molecules and chemicals. None take into account the whole person, so I needed to dig more deeply, exploring perspectives that see cancer as a result of stress or unresolved emotional or spiritual conflicts. So, again, we must ask the question ... *what is cancer?*

Wilhelm Reich, an Austrian psychoanalyst of the generation after Freud, observed that when there is sexual dysfunction, the body loses vitality and we become emotionally imbalanced, which alters cellular metabolism and eventually causes cancer. To Reich, cancer is systemic—a condition of the person as a whole.[13]

He was the first contemporary researcher to see that cancer can be based on emotional distress, and he inspired others to follow the thread of a mind-body imbalance or disorder. The founders of many systems of bodywork and other human potential modalities followed suit. Alexander Lowen, father of bioenergetics, and Fritz Perls, who developed gestalt therapy, both explored ways the personality is reflected in the body and especially (Lowen) in the ways we move. Their perspectives address, among other things, the muscular armor we develop to adapt to experiences that feel unsafe.

The relation between psyche and biology was also explored by the German physician Ryke Geerd Hamer, who noted that Reich's insights were by no means new, that in fact for millennia men and women have recognized the psychic origins of illness. He refers to cancer as **an adaptive biological response** to trauma, rather than as an illness. According to Hamer, when the *shock* is resolved, the body returns to normal.

Some researchers who agree with Hamer's thesis that cancer is an adaptive response explain how neoplasticity, the capacity to produce new tissue, as is the case with cancer, might create more evolved beings able to survive a stressful environment.[14] Hypermutation, some think, might be an attempt to produce a **more evolved cellular structure.**

Some other researchers theorize that cancer **is a result of a spiritual disconnect** or a call to connect with life's meaning. Analytical psychiatrist

Carl Gustav Jung regarded a life with meaning as a prerequisite of health.

The way we think about cancer, i.e., the metaphor we use to describe cancer, colors our response, how we cope with it, and the way we face treatment.

Cancer as an Elephant

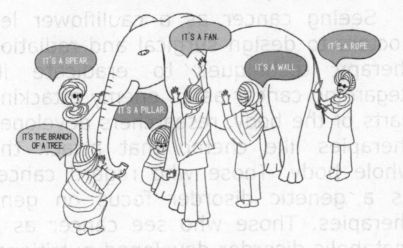

Cancer as an elephant.

The Buddha told a story about six blind men who were asked to describe an elephant by touching different parts of its body.

Each man touched a different place on the elephant, and then they argued for a long time about what it was they had touched. Every man maintained his own opinion, which became stronger and more rigid over time, and they couldn't reach agreement. Each had his own point of view, and only when they opened to aggregating their perspectives were they able to know the elephant as a whole.

Seeing cancer as a cauliflower led doctors to design surgical and radiation therapy techniques to eradicate it. Regarding cancer as an enemy attacking parts of the body, researchers developed therapies like chemo that attack the whole body. Those who regard cancer as a genetic disorder focus on gene therapies. Those who see cancer as a metabolic disorder developed nutritional therapies along with vitamin and mineral supplements. Explaining cancer as a result of emotional distress, we engage psychological and somatic psychotherapies. In cultures where cancer is considered a consequence of possession, people turn to exorcists, priests, and healing masses.

Each model is based on a perspective. Like the blind men and the elephant, each perspective probably offers a part of the truth, and it's necessary to consider them all to have an overview of the conditions that brought about a cancer diagnosis.

One thing all these models share is the perspective that cancer is caused by cells growing autonomously and out of control, invading other tissues locally or remotely. In fact, this description does not match reality and leaves a host of unanswered questions.

We speak about cancer *as an invader,* even though we know it doesn't exactly come from the outside. Within a single family carrying a mutated gene predisposing an entire generation to certain types of cancer, some family members get it and others don't. Not all cancer cells circulating in our blood metastasize.[16] Two people suffering from the same cancer show radically different patterns of evolution; one might be cured and the other not. What are the critical variables? Does it depend on the cancer or the person's response?

How Does the Mind Function?

First we frame a picture of the way we believe things are, and then we live within that framework. Whatever does not fit within that framework is referred to as mystery: inexplicable, nonsensical, or perhaps supernatural.

—Longchenpa, *Now That I Come to Die*[15]

Science is similar. Theories purport to explain phenomena until more comprehensive theories appear. This is how science advances.

To answer this, we need to look beyond what we call cancer and focus on the person. *So, then, what is cancer?* After reflecting on all these models, I was able to provide Carolina with an integrative response.

Cancer is a multifactorial disease, more than a genetic, metabolic disorder, more than a psychological, emotional, or spiritual imbalance. Autopsies of people who have died in accidents or "from old age" show a high percentage of undiagnosed tumors.[17] And some tumors disappear with no observable treatment at all.[18] We produce small tumors all the time that our immune system destroys or keeps under control, and they remain unnoticed throughout our lives.

A clinical study on women with breast cancer confirmed that by treating the bones, metastasis was prevented. After surgery, radiation, and/or chemotherapy, these women were treated with zoledronic acid, a substance used for fortifying bones. It has no known direct anticancer effect. In fact, it's usually prescribed to prevent or treat osteoporosis. In this study, it was used to treat the *field,* i.e., the bones, one of the common places to which breast cancer metastasizes. By treating the field without any further anticancer treatment, the number of women developing bone metastasis diminished.[19] Until then, the only acceptable treatments for metastasis were those with direct anticancer effects, like hormones or chemotherapy. In this study, it was proven that by strengthening the field (the bones), metastasis was prevented, suggesting that metastasis depends not only on the cancer, but also on the host field.

Recent research is prompting a paradigm shift that is widening our understanding of cancer. Seeing it as a group of cells growing autonomously is only part of the picture, like looking at the hands of a watch without taking into account the numerals in the background.

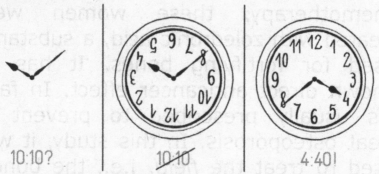

10:10?   10:10   4:40!

It is the context that gives meaning.

The figure-ground set represents a whole, or *gestalt.* In an experimental psychology lab in Germany in the early twentieth century, it was shown that the human mind organizes perceptions as shapes and entireties (gestalts). When we look at a flower in a meadow, we perceive qualities like color, shape, and texture, and also the plants that surround it. We perceive the flower and the meadow as a coherent whole. If we pick the flower and put it in a vase at home, our perception will be different, not because the flower has changed, but because the flower-environment entirety has changed. In sculpture or ceramics, the *figure-ground relationship* produces either contrast, or if the object and its background are similar, a merge.

Focusing *only* on cancer cells is like focusing only on the figure. Cancer cannot exist without a background, a system supporting its existence. What we have been calling cancer is the active part within the whole that appears to have become autonomous.

PNIE Network

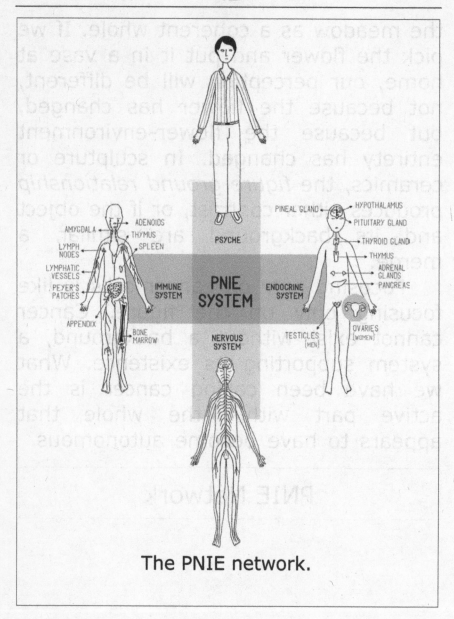

The PNIE network.

What we call the immune system is part of a wider internal intelligence network known as the psycho-neuro-immuno-endocrine network (PNIE, abbreviated sometimes as PNI, PENI, or PNEI).[20] This is the *ground* that needs to be a part of our perception. When the immune system and the PNIE network give way to abnormal, invasive cells, cancer spreads. These abnormal cells depend on this background, which is no less active than the malignant cells themselves.

When we consider cancer as a whole, we can redefine the disease process and expand the approach to treatment.

Whether a tumor or mass of cells (the figure) continues to spread depends in part on its and our response arising from the immune system and the PNIE network (the ground, or host). This integrative approach recognizes the contribution of the PNIE network and thus allows seeing the whole, the significance of the figure *and* the ground. To have a full picture, we must see both.

According to the new health-disease model, based mainly on the psycho-neuro-immuno-endocrinology (PNIE) approach, cancer can be defined as a disease caused by the uncontrolled proliferation of a group of cells *in a body with an immune system and a PNIE network that allows them to invade other tissues wildly—locally and at a distance—and that without treatment can lead to death.*

This integrative approach leads us to focus not only on the cancer treatment, but also on how to positively affect the host and its PNIE intelligence network to help it control the cancer and sometimes even to revert it. Genetic, metabolic, emotional, spiritual, and mental factors affect the PNIE network.

By taking into account different points of view, like the blind people in the story, we can understand the elephant in its wholeness and seek combined strategies that consider the human as a multidimensional being[21] with a body, mind, emotions, spirit, and social context. These strategies will include healthy habits—nutrition, exercise, and sleep, restoring emotional balance, and spiritual reconnection to positively affect the PNIE intelligence network that for so many decades knew how to maintain our health and allow it to play the main role again.

It is important to keep each part of the elephant in mind in order to understand cancer as:

the manifestation

of a global imbalance in a multidimensional human being,

in which, in presence of a breakdown in the immune system and PNIE network, allows a group of cells

to develop a hypermutation condition and metabolic disorder,

to start growing in an abnormal and uncontrolled way,

and eventually, to invade the body and lead to death.

This is why cancer, though located in only one organ, is an illness that affects the whole person and not just the affected organ. Hence, the treatment should, from the very beginning, focus on the whole person.

Take-Home Message

In developed countries, 50 percent of cancers are cured.

The word *cancer* represents hundreds of different diseases.

The causes of cancer are usually multifactorial.

Which metaphor we use to describe the disease defines how we cope with it and how we face the treatment.

Positive changes in lifestyle reduce the risk of cancer and help recover health.

Cancer is an illness that affects the person as a whole.

Each host, each person's cancer case, is unique.

Chapter 3

WHY DO WE GET SICK?

All things break. And all things can be mended. Not with time, as they say, but with intention. So, go. Love intentionally, extravagantly, unconditionally. The broken world waits in darkness for the light that is you.

—L.R. KNOST

Claudio, an active trader from a small town, came to me for a second opinion. He had a long medical history. As a child, he'd had a benign tumor removed, and ten years later, he developed diabetes and coronary heart disease, requiring two stents.[1] Now he'd been diagnosed with a lymphoma. "Why do I get sick so often?" he asked, worried and confused.

The way we live affects our health. I explained that if we eat processed, nutrient-deficient foods, don't exercise, suffer from sleep disorder, accumulate stress,[2] don't process emotions, use harmful substances like nicotine, or don't find meaning in our lives, our health is affected.

Persistent, unhealthy conditions like these overload the PNIE network, preventing it from maintaining the internal balance necessary for optimal health. When the PNIE network becomes overloaded, the immune system can't always give full attention to important, even urgent, demands, including disease.

I listened carefully to Claudio's story, asking him about his life, trying to understand why he got sick so often. Claudio couldn't understand why I asked certain questions, like whether he liked his job. He said he was stressed about work, "like everybody." I explained that stress could be an imbalance between a demand and our ability to meet it.

We all have an involuntary nervous system—also called the autonomic nervous system—that regulates the functioning of our internal organs. This system consists of an accelerator (sympathetic nervous system) and a brake (parasympathetic or vagotonic nervous system). When demands arise in everyday life, even demanding thoughts like "I have to...," it's like stepping on the gas. When we take five minutes to relax from the daily hustle and bustle, it's like easing your foot on the brake.

Both the accelerator and the brake are needed for everyday life. To live in balance, we need to alternate between having our foot on the gas and easing on the brake. If we only step on the gas, our system becomes unbalanced, and we're unable to react appropriately to each situation.

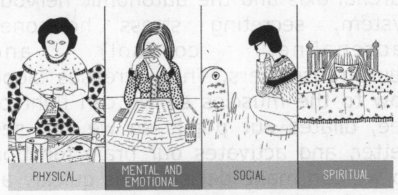

| PHYSICAL | MENTAL AND EMOTIONAL | SOCIAL | SPIRITUAL |

Factors that affect health.

What Does It Mean to "Mobilize Energy"?

> Before lifting weights, we take a deep breath and hold it. This is a way of mobilizing energy.

Our response to stress, or threats, is the same as our ancestors had. When a predator appeared, they stood and faced the danger or they ran away—fight or flight. In moments like these, the body instantly increases energy, strength, and power so we can run, shout, or defend ourselves.

The stress response affects the psycho-neuro-immuno-endocrine system by activating the hypothalamic-pituitary-adrenal axis and the autonomic nervous system, secreting stress hormones (adrenaline, cortisol) and neurotransmitters. This increases blood flow to the muscles so we can fight or flee, dilates our pupils so we can see better, and activates our brain function so we can make decisions as quickly as possible. The immune, digestive, and reproductive systems are deactivated so full attention can be directed toward the danger at hand.

Facing a stressful situation, our body automatically steps on the gas, triggering a response to mobilize energy in the presence of danger. The PNIE system is stimulated, and stress hormones—adrenaline and cortisol—are released.

Practice for Healthy Living

Jump up and down fifteen times. Then put your hand on your chest, feel your heart, and listen to your breathing. This feeling is the same as when the acute stress response is activated.

The acute stress response can be life-saving when we're faced with a threat, as when we cross the street without paying attention and a vehicle comes barreling toward us. We need to react immediately to avoid being run over. **When our stress response is activated, even if the trigger is habitual or imagined, our internal alert reaction is the same.** A shock like the threat of losing our job or relationship problems triggers the same biological reaction.

When the stress response is activated, the body will react in some way and discharge the energy that has been mobilized. Then, when the threat is over, the body will go into a relaxation period, so hormonal levels can recover. When a dog hears a strange sound, it runs outside, discharges its adrenaline by barking, and then comes back, lies down, and returns to relaxation.

Practice for Healthy Living

Take time every day to release energy.

Exercise regularly.

Explore meditation, yoga, and other stress-release methods to promote internal balance.

"Now I see why you're asking about my life, but how can I know when I'm accumulating adrenaline?" asked Claudio.

I explained that detecting acute stress can be easy; you only have to listen to your body. Palpitations, quickened breathing, and sweaty palms are signals of energy mobilization, showing that the stress response is activated.

Practice for Healthy Living

Think about the dog discharging its adrenaline so it can relax again. Now do the same. Search for a way to discharge that energy. Go for a walk, do some exercise, listen to music, scream, kick, or dance. Release the stress from your body.

I continued to explain to Claudio that the problem begins when we don't discharge that adrenaline in everyday life. We feel frozen before certain situations or repress our desire to discharge what we feel inside. The energy we've mobilized stays stuck inside and produces stress signals, such as insomnia, irritability, inability to concentrate, anger, or annoyance.

Which of the Following Might Be Anxiety-Producing for You?

• The **novelty** of learning to use a new computer or a new phone, or expecting your first child.

> • The **uncertainty** of whether your child's babysitter will arrive on time so you can go to work, or whether your volatile boss will be in a good or bad mood.
>
> • The **threat** to your ego when your child's teacher asks if you spend enough time with your child, or when a new employee asks a million questions to challenge your competency.
>
> • The **loss of control** when something is stolen, or when you're stuck in traffic and realize you won't arrive at your appointment on time.

It's important to identify *situations that stress us,* ones that make us NUTS. They usually have one or more of these characteristics:

N = New, novel

U = Unexpected, unpredictable

T = Threat to our ego

S = Sense of being out of control

When the adrenaline rush fails to discharge after the stressor has passed, and it happens again and again, we begin to experience chronic stress.

Keeping tension bottled up inside is exhausting and makes it hard to continue facing life. Stress has three stages:[3] alarm (acute stress), resistance (continued stress), and exhaustion (chronic stress). During the acute stage, we feel revved up, but anxious. Once we start to develop resistance and exhaustion, we might feel hostile or depressed.

"I agree with you, Doctor. I face many of these things. My father has been in a vegetative state for years, suffering from advanced Alzheimer's disease. We have financial difficulties, uncertain how long we can afford his medical expenses, not to mention the stress having to bear this situation. You're also right when you say stress shows up as anger. I become aggressive with my wife, and I've lost enthusiasm even for the things I used to love, like fishing or spending time with my friends. And I feel exhausted 24/7. A lot of people I know are stressed but never get sick. Why me?" Claudio asked.

I explained that something that stresses one person might not stress another. It depends on attitude and many other factors. If you're affected negatively by a situation, it can manifest as a symptom. You can feel threatened by an increase in demands or a reduction of resources or the thought about what you "should" be doing. Demands can be external: traffic, work, finances, conflicts, or even information overload. Demands can also be internal. Sometimes we feel under pressure even when we're not undergoing a stressful situation on the outside. The anticipation of a threatening situation, whether it occurs or not, can cause the release of stress hormones.

Anticipating an event can be worse than the event itself. When we perseverate about a situation, spending hours thinking about it, we secrete stress hormones, and this chronic release of hormones affects our health negatively. Chronically elevated cortisol levels inhibit the immune system and diminish the body's ability to defend and repair itself. Thus, a stress response depends not only on the external situation, but also on the way we perceive it and our response.

> *People are not disturbed by things, but by the view they take of them.*
>
> —EPICTETUS

The brain is like a powerful central processing unit (CPU) of a computer that controls and coordinates our activities, translating external experiences to inner operating instructions. Sense organs receive external signals and transmit them to the brain where, together with memories of things past, the mind *perceives* what is happening. The brain is the *hardware,* and the mind is the *software.*

The Rope and the Snake

You are in a dark lane at twilight and you see an awkward snake on the floor before you.

Suddenly, somebody comes from the other side and, while he walks beside the snake, asks you why you are scared.

> *You tell him everything about that poisonous snake which they have almost come across.*
>
> *Then he answers you, and shows you that it is only a rope.*
>
> *The snake doesn't exist, but, however, with the power of illusion and superimposition, the notion of snake may hide the rope, the reality.*[4]
> —Papaji

Indian philosophy talks about *maya* or illusion. The snake is maya, a distorted perception of reality. If we think the snake is real, we are afraid and we suffer. Beyond the veils of illusion, we see that it is a rope. That is the ultimate reality.

Every time our mind interprets a situation and sends messages to the whole body through the PNIE network using hormones and neurotransmitters, it modifies the inner landscape. The PNIE network and the immune response are agents of an intelligence system that sends information to the smallest corners of the body, the cellular level, about the environment and life conditions. What is transmitted, then, is not "truth," but what we perceive. **Our mind creates our reality.**

> *It is not seeing that makes us believe, but believing that enables us to see.*
> —JUAN ANTONIO BAYONA, DIRECTOR, *THE ORPHANAGE* (2007)

If we are expecting a phone call from our son because he is late, and we're worried that he might have had an accident, we bring this into our body. We feel anxiety and anguish and produce stress substances and alert signals. If we think he isn't calling us because he's having a good time at a party, we relax, and our body produces wellness substances.

"It's true," admitted Claudio. *"I spend a lot of time feeling anxious about things that never happen."*

I explained to him that continuous anxiety, in the long term, makes us sick, and I explained how it happens. **Becoming aware of what's happening is the first step in bringing about change.**

The mind is like a washing machine with two settings: **calm** and **alert.** If it believes our situation is safe, it transmits through the PNIE network that this is a time for the organs to replenish and repair tissues. This is how we nourish ourselves, recover from illnesses, and reproduce ourselves. If the mind believes we're threatened, it will message the body to take care only of urgent matters.

We Are a Walking Pharmacy

We produce wellness or stress substances, according to our perceptions of the environment and the meaning we give to our experiences.

At least 30 percent of patients experience the effects of a medicine, or even a surgery, without receiving the actual medicine or procedure. This is the "placebo effect."[5]

It is produced by the activation of internal substances, our "internal pharmacy," which act on the same pain receptors as medicines do. Many medicines are, in fact, simply copies of substances we produce by ourselves.[6]

Both responses—calm and alert—are reflected in the PNIE network and, as a result, in the body's immune response. It's important to understand how our state of mind affects each cell of our body, through hormones, neurotransmitters, and other information molecules. *Information molecules* is a comprehensive term that refers to all substances that carry information within the psychological, neurological, immune, and endocrine systems. They include neurotransmitters, immunomodulators, and hormones, among others. We used to think that neurotransmitters carried information only within the nervous system. Now we know they're also produced by other systems, such as the digestive system. The term *information molecules* includes all substances that function within a system and connect different systems.

Our thoughts are translated into our biology.

Buddhists train their minds so they function in service to the person. In the West, most people's minds are not trained, and when we get triggered, a cacophony of thoughts can echo uncontrollably within. Repetitive images, memories, and concerns play over and over, arousing fear and anxiety and keeping the body on continuous alert.[7]

Two Monks and a Woman

Two monks met a beautiful woman at a riverbank. Like them, she wanted to cross the river, but she was staring at the water in fear. One of the monks decided to help, and he carried her across the river.

The other monk was upset but said nothing. Buddhist monks take a vow not to touch women, and his companion had not only touched her, but had carried her in his arms.

After a long walk back to the monastery, the angry monk blurted out, "I will tell our master what you've done!"

The other monk asked, "What are you talking about?"

"You carried that beautiful young lady across the river."

"Oh," said the monk being accused. "I left her on the riverbank. It seems you're still carrying her."[8]

If we're always on alert, our **system will inevitably fail.** Do you remember when cars had chokes, like motorcycles, to adjust the ratio of gasoline to air? If you leave the choke on all the time, eventually the engine will fail from overwork—too much fuel. When we're under chronic stress, the system begins to flash a warning light, but usually we adopt behavioral patterns that only compound the problem. We smoke, drink, abuse substances, overeat, and enter toxic relationships (power struggles, rage, victimization), searching for satisfaction but really for an escape from the discomfort (imbalance) we're feeling. The situation only worsens because a feedback system, difficult to get out of, is in place. **Chronic stress is a primary cause of unwellness in modern life.**

When we're stressed, we interpret ordinary signals as alarm bells. The story of the rope and the snake is an example of misinterpreting a situation and suffering because of it.

On a Day-to-Day Basis, Do You See Ropes or Snakes?

When a jealous person sees or hears something, a grand drama arises in his or her mind. A stubborn person sees through the lens of stubbornness and gets into unnecessary arguments.

How many times do we misunderstand, hearing something that isn't said or seeing something that isn't there?

We receive information from the external world through our senses, but we interpret according to past experiences and conditioning. Our perceptions are often far from reality. Misperceptions get us into arguments, and we suffer.

> Only when we calm our mind can we see more clearly. Only then do the ghosts fade.

"Thank you, Laura, but how does this relate to cancer?" Claudio asked.

In earlier days, our ancestors knew that chronically stressed and depressed people get sick more frequently. Today, science shows us how chronic stress and depression affect our immunity, making us more vulnerable to diseases like cancer. We've already seen that a mutated cell will proliferate and form a tumor when the environment is conducive. Current research focuses on cell mutiny as well as background conditions. A tumor exists in a "community" that includes cancer cells, normal cells, and the immune system's cells, which are messengers of the PNIE system mounting a response to the cancer cells. The coexisting populations in this microenvironment determine whether the cancer cells are killed, proliferate locally, or invade and metastasize widely. In situations of stress, normal cells become senescent, which means they stop reproducing and turn immortal. At the beginning, this mechanism can be protective and prevent cancer. But if senescent cells don't die, in the long run they produce inflammatory substances that, in the tumor microenvironment, promote cancer.[9]

How Cancer Grows

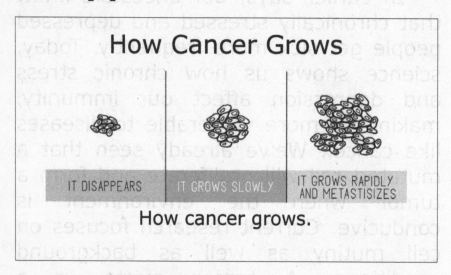

IT DISAPPEARS   IT GROWS SLOWLY   IT GROWS RAPIDLY AND METASTISIZES

How cancer grows.

Cells Can Survive in Two Ways

When external conditions are favorable, cells reproduce themselves. When external conditions are unfavorable, cells can become autonomous and immortal, i.e., malignant.[10] Such a metaphor for cancer! How are *your* external conditions—your relationships, your workplace? How are your internal conditions? How do you treat yourself? Are you overly demanding? What do you do when things don't work out the way you'd hoped?

Pivotal is how the mind perceives what is happening, how that's translated through the PNIE network, and what information arrives at the tumor microenvironment. If the mind is chronically on alert, as when we're in a bad relationship or reliving a trauma from childhood or military service, the PNIE network's urgency systems can be triggered, placing priority on responding to stressors engendered by our thoughts, and they might fail to recognize mutated cells to stop their uncontrolled growth.

How We Translate Our Experiences Internally

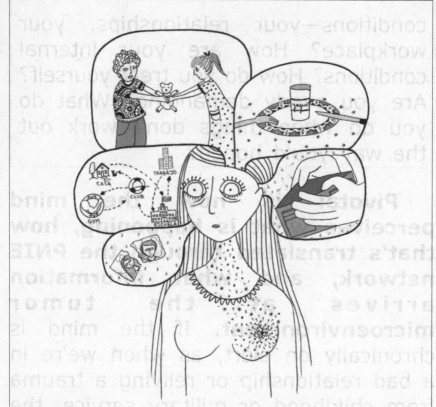

How we translate our experiences internally.

"We're under a lot of stress brought about by my father's illness. But we've always been a rigid family; I had a strict, authoritarian upbringing. My sister became an addict. On top of this, we were ripped off by another branch of our family," continued Claudio.

Together, Claudio and I reviewed a series of experiences that led him to live in chronic stress—surgeries, work, financial and family demands, violent relationships, self-demands, and fraud. Now it was easier to recognize how Claudio felt so vulnerable and how the demands on him exceeded his resources. At first, he'd been able to cope, but finally the accumulation of stressors weakened him, and he wasn't able to deal with them all. I explained that when energy disperses in so many directions, not much is left to invest in the body. The same happens to the immune system; when it's overloaded with work, it has nothing left to maintain our health.

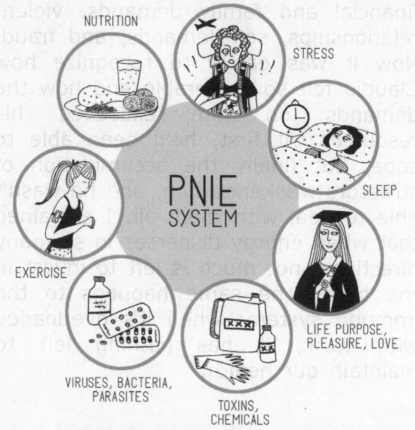

NUTRITION

STRESS

SLEEP

PNIE
SYSTEM

EXERCISE

LIFE PURPOSE,
PLEASURE, LOVE

VIRUSES, BACTERIA,
PARASITES

TOXINS,
CHEMICALS

What affects the PNIE system.

Some people associate cancer development with a contentious divorce or the death of a loved one. Generally, these events represent the last straw of a system already on chronic alert—overloaded and overworking. In that internal environment, one more significant stressor can cause the immune system and the PNIE network to break down, unable to cope. This process takes time; it doesn't happen overnight.

The systems-view paradigm invites us to abandon linear thinking—a single cause for a single effect, or in this case a single factor developing a single cancer.[11] It isn't a mathematical equation where A+B=C. **The causes of cancer are usually multifactorial** and different for each person. In some people, a combination of unhealthy diet, divorce, and losing a job might develop a cancer, while in others it doesn't. It also depends on our resources, the tools we can call upon to face challenges.

What Makes the System Fail?

Even though the imbalance might appear in the form of a tumor in an organ, cancer is the representation of a global system imbalance, or failure, that may have been produced by some or all of the following factors:
- physical factors: e.g., eating disorders, sedentary lifestyle
- mental-emotional factors: e.g., chronic stress, depression

> • social factors: e.g., contentious divorce, death of a loved one
> • spiritual factors: e.g., loss of meaning in life, loss of aspiration, loss of desire

Looking for the stressor that put a person out of balance is not to blame the person or the stressor. Most important is to help us take responsibility for our own health and to be true to ourselves.

We're beginning to see that **cancer is a complex manifestation of a systemic failure,** the result of the progression of physiopathological processes that interweave with genetic, environmental, behavioral, psychological, and social factors that help the newly emerging mutated cells acquire the ability to proliferate, invade, and stimulate the *angiogenesis* (formation of new arteries that feed the cancer cells) until they become malignant. This process develops through an exchange between cancer cells and their microenvironment, and inflammation plays a leading role in facilitating tumor growth and metastasis, or not.

Inflammation is a biological response to harmful stimuli, such as bacteria, damaged cells, or introduced chemicals. In an effort to kill foreign bacteria and prevent the damage from spreading, the body recruits the cells of the immune system (leukocytes, or white blood cells) and produces blood vessels and other molecules of information. This is why the area becomes red, hot, and painful. When the threat passes, the inflammatory reaction normally subsides. In some diseases, though, like arthritis, the immune system triggers an inflammatory response even when there are no foreign invaders to fight off. The body's normally protective immune system begins to damage its own tissues, engendering an autoimmune disease.

When a cancer cell is detected, the immune system might respond in different ways. If the response is pro-inflammatory, the cells and information molecules produced may actually encourage the cancer to grow. We can no longer see cancer as something that happened to us. As with an autoimmune disease, cancer is showing that the immune system as it is can no longer function properly and, although by a different mechanism, may even be promoting "disease."

There Are No Illnesses, Only People Who Get Sick

In the late nineteenth century, two important French scientists researched the causes of illness and postulated contrary theories. Claude Bernard studied physiology and argued that disease is caused by a weak host, or terrain. Louis Pasteur discovered the role of microbes as the cause of infectious diseases such as tuberculosis, which at that time were the main causes of death. Near the end of his life, Pasteur recognized, "Bernard was right. The microbe is nothing, the terrain is everything." Microbes will only cause and develop a disease in a fertile terrain.

Once cancer has appeared, a system in failure expressed by the constant activation of the hypothalamic-pituitary-adrenal axis contributes to a fertile microenvironment for the suppression of the immune system, growth of tumor cells, stimulation of invasion and migration, and angiogenesis. Some authors suggest that cancer is a *verb* rather than a noun. It emerges as a manifestation of a system's failure and remains unless the conditions change. Danny Hillis, in his TED Talk, said:

> I think we're even wrong when we talk about cancer as a thing. This is the big mistake. I think cancer should not be a noun. We should talk about *cancering* as something we do, not something we have. And so tumors are symptoms of cancer. And your body is probably cancering all the time. But there are lots of systems in your body that keep it under control.[12]

Claudio was becoming interested in achieving a healthier way of life. He kept analyzing the disease process and bringing up new concerns. One day, while we were talking on Skype, he posed a challenging question, "Laura, it seems clear that many people who suffer from cancer have pretty messy lives. But Josefina, my thirty-three-year-old niece, has just been diagnosed with ovarian cancer, and she leads a peaceful life. How do you explain this?"

I repeated to Claudio that our mind is trained to think in a linear fashion: one cause for one effect. We were raised this way, but it's not actually useful for understanding cancer or many of the complex things that happen to us. Though two people may develop the same illness, each case might be a consequence of different factors. Thus, the illness is not the problem; it's a signal showing us that the life we're leading isn't serving us anymore. Life is constantly encouraging us to develop more complex ways of thinking.

It was difficult for me to find out what the illness was manifesting in the case of Josefina without knowing her. What had made her ill? What was happening in her life?

It is much more important to know what sort of a patient has a disease;

than what sort of a disease a patient has.

—WILLIAM OSLER

As we saw in the last chapter, "So ... What Is Cancer?" we are multidimensional human beings, with bodies, minds, emotions, and spirits in a social context. *Most failures arise at the mind-body-emotion level*—we haven't taken good care of ourselves; we have unresolved conflicts, especially in relationships; we impose excessive demands; we don't fully understand what's happening to us.

But the failure, or warning, *may come from the spiritual dimension.* It's not unusual to hear about someone getting ill from sadness. After a spouse's death, for example, a husband might not want to live any longer and prefer to go with his beloved. In the same way, we meet people whose lives have somehow lost meaning, and they become sick. This is why we have to explore each person as a single, unique human being. Josefina's cancer could be seen, rather than as a systemic failure, as a warning that the life she's leading does not meet her needs as a bio-psycho-social-spiritual human being.

Cancer is an alarm system showing that something must be changed. It is an expression of our survival instinct responding to conditions that threaten our physical health or take us away from meaning in our life. In this way, **cancer is a demand for change.**

Take-Home Message

The life we lead affects our health. Chronic stress is a primary cause of disease.

Reality is shaped by the way our mind perceives it. Our thoughts directly affect our body.

We are a walking pharmacy.

Cancer is a manifestation of the system failure, regarding conditions that threaten our physical health or separate us from the meaning of our life.

Cancer is a call to change. The first step is to become aware of the life we are leading.

Chapter 4

NOW WHAT?

In that inevitable, excruciatingly human moment, we are offered a powerful choice. Will we interpret this loss as so unjust, unfair, and devastating—or will we somehow feel this loss as an opportunity to become more tender, more open, more passionately alive?
—WAYNE MULLER[1]

Mirta, a sixty-five-year-old psychologist who had been diagnosed with lung cancer, came to see me. She had been a heavy smoker until ten years earlier and was unable to understand why she was getting cancer now. I explained that thinking in a linear way, "Smoking causes cancer," prevents us from seeing the whole system. If reality were linear, why do some smokers get cancer while others don't? Why had Mirta been healthy until now? What changed that allowed cancer to appear?

There are many variables, including the ways emotions impact our immune system. Understanding this can empower us to make healthier choices and relieve us of guilt for past decisions. When we are ready to act on new information, we can be grateful and proactive. Feeling guilty for not acting sooner is not helpful and can delay us from acting on our own behalf.

When cancer appears, something in the system is breaking down, and this co-creates the field where cancer cells appear, activate, and proliferate. We're dynamic, complex systems formed by interconnected, interwoven elements.[2] Emergent qualities appear from interactions among the parts that cannot be explained by any single element alone. I told Mirta that cancer is not an "enemy" attacking from the outside. It's a systemic manifestation of who we are today, as a bio-psycho-social-spiritual being. Smoking in the past was certainly a factor, but other factors had to be present also.[3] It wasn't a question of feeling guilty for having smoked, but an opportunity to learn what else, besides the cigarettes, could be detrimental to our health that we need to change.

We have a physical body and an energetic body, and the latter can be further divided into our emotional, mental, and spiritual dimensions. (See chapter 7, "The Treasure Hunt.") We act as though they are separate; that makes it easier for our linear thought processes to understand. But they are elements of a whole that in fact cannot be separated from one another. A change in one dimension produces changes throughout the system. For example, drinking six cups of coffee (physical dimension) can produce hyperstimulation and anxiety (mental dimension) and even aggression (emotional dimension).

In addition, we're part of families and social groups that are also complex, dynamic systems. All dimensions are connected and affect one another. A wedding (social dimension), for example, brings happiness (emotional dimension) to many members of the family. Each level of this system is part of something even more complex. A cell is part of an organ, which is part of a system (e.g., digestive), which is part of a human being, which is part of a family, a nation, and the human race.

Although we can describe each level of this complex system, we cannot predict exactly how any one element will function on a linear basis. As a result of the interactions among parts, new emergent properties appear that cannot be explained by or attributed to the properties of any single part. The interaction of multiple dimensions results in something new, not just a modification of one or more of the parts. Weather, for example, is a complex system. Meteorologists may know the winds, tides, and temperature, but they cannot predict with 100 percent certainty if it's going to rain and at what time. A prediction about the course of a disease is as uncertain as predicting the weather.

Mirta and I applied these concepts to her case. Her diagnosis had terrified her and represented a deep concern and sorrow for her whole family. Conversely, family problems can lead to imbalances that affect our health.

When a system is out of balance, a failure on one level affects the whole.

When a failure arises on the social or family level and the mind cannot equilibrate the imbalance, the body might act as a messenger and the imbalance might show up as an illness. In such cases, treatment needs to be global and not just addressing the affected organ. Treating the body in isolation would not address the imbalance in the whole system.

Because she'd smoked for years, Mirta had a predisposition to lung cancer. As long as her immune system and psycho-neuro-immuno-endocrine (PNIE) response were working well, she was healthy. But health is influenced by many factors, including the way we take care of our body, the way we process stress, and the way we relate to others.

"Okay," she said. "I understand that the problem is not just in my lungs, but what do we do now?"

If we consider that cancer is a manifestation at the level of an organ, telling us something about that human being as a whole—and moreover, about the social group of which she is a part—there might be multiple factors at different levels leading to a continuous breakdown of the system.

Two people traveling in Cleveland will each have a distinct experience. One drives; the other flies. Although they both end up in Cleveland, what and how brings each of them there is different. And to get back home, each will have to take a different path appropriate to needs and circumstances. Two people, although they have the same type and stage of cancer, arrived there through different combinations of unhealthy factors, so each has a unique road back to good health. The treatment will be custom-tailored according to what has been making each of them sick.

Integrative oncology helps each person identify the factors that might be stressing their system. A personalized approach is necessary to find the guiding thread to undo the factors that took us to our disease and to finding the way out.

Many Authors Compare Disease to a Journey

A journey of a thousand miles begins with a single step.
—Laozi

Mirta's recovery plan included conventional medicine to remove her tumors and treatments and practices that could help repair her system's failure and guide her back to health. She affirmed that recovery was her priority, and she was ready to begin her journey.

I suggested she begin by setting aside time each day for self-care, focusing on her health and recovering her balance. When unhealthy lifestyle choices—physical, emotional, social, or spiritual—lead to disease, the task is to reverse the conditions and re-create a way of life that restores and sustains health. Turning around lifestyle habits requires will and intention and is difficult when the body is depleted. It's important to **begin by moving the stagnant energy that has**

accumulated in the body or replenishing it if it has depleted.

Mirta felt exhausted. She needed to learn to discern what nourished her from what drained her energy, not just during physical exertion but during conversations and other exchanges of energy throughout the day.

We reviewed what seemed to "fill her tank." Walking in the park and sharing an enjoyable movie with a loved one were replenishing for her. She was interested in Reiki, and I encouraged her to do that, and to choose among other activities to see who and what was energizing and to include these in her weekly plan.

It was also important for her to recognize what drained her energy. There are people who leave us exhausted after talking with them, and activities like waiting in line at the bank or shopping in a crowded supermarket can make us feel tired and moody. It can help to have fewer of these activities or to do them differently. For example, listening to music while waiting in line can make the experience more enjoyable and increase our energy.

Practice for Healthy Living

What nourishes me?
What drains my energy?
Write it down.

Physical exertion can help move stagnant energy. Walking at least thirty minutes several times a week brings energy back into circulation. Reflexology, acupuncture, or energy healing can also be helpful.

The parents of Daniel, a sixteen-year-old boy, asked if I would visit him in the hospital. Daniel had had chest pains for several months. At first, they thought it was related to his soccer practice. Then he started feeling exhausted and losing weight, and a more thorough exam showed he had a Ewing sarcoma on one of his ribs. The cancer was potentially curable, but it would be costly. Treatment would last at least six months—first, aggressive chemotherapy; then surgery; and perhaps at the end, a bone marrow transplant. It was a frightening prognosis for a boy who until then had been thinking only about soccer and partying.

Daniel and I had a long conversation. I explained that he was undergoing something much bigger than he'd been told. I compared it to an adventure and said his attitude would be critically important. He found my words hard to understand.

"Laura, you're saying this is an adventure, but I'm confined within these four walls!" he told me, frustrated and angry. I acknowledged that this way of seeing was unfamiliar, especially when you're confined to a room and everyone else is talking about battling an illness. "The most important thing," I said, "is to show up. It's the same as when you play a strong opponent in soccer. If you have a good attitude and, at the same time, do all you can to enjoy it, you and your team will fare better. **When we can't change a situation, we can change our attitude.**"[4]

Daniel needed to **focus on something pleasant** to boost his immunity. Possibilities included watching funny movies, talking with friends on

Skype, reading or having someone read inspiring stories to him, and some creative activity. Daniel had wanted to learn to play guitar for a long time. It seemed an excellent idea. He also wanted to make a photo album. For the next few months he was going to have a lot of time, and it was a good idea to focus on activities that would nourish his soul.

We also talked about the **importance of seeking help.** Many people don't like asking for help, and some barely know how to. Disease offers a chance to cultivate this capacity. Those with cancer often need help with chores they find tiring or cumbersome, such as shopping so they can eat healthily. They might also lack a companion for walks and support to engage in healthful activities.

In almost every hero's journey, the protagonist has a companion, someone or a team to encourage and accompany that person along the way. I encouraged Daniel to think about forming a team.

Practice for Healthy Living

Ask someone to go to the supermarket for you.

Go to the bank with someone and ask that person to wait in line and call you when it's your turn.

Ask a friend to find some comedy movies and watch them together.

"It's like when you went river rafting and chose the people you wanted to come with you," I told him. "And you get to decide how you'd like each person to help you. They can sit at the front or the back of the raft. You choose who you want to paddle and who you'd like to navigate the rapids."

His parents, offering him love and daily support, would be in the raft with him. He also chose a guitar teacher, one sister to help with the photo album, and his other sister to select funny movies they could watch together. As time went on, he added an uncle to accompany him on walks and a few classmates to help him keep up with schoolwork. Daniel selected his team brilliantly, according to his needs.

As time progressed, his mother reached her wit's end and slowed down, looked for help, and focused on herself and her own well-being as well. Caregiving can be very demanding, and it's important for caregivers to practice self-care, too. When she did this, Daniel had to expand and renew his team.

"A couple of friends come to visit," he told me, *"and we laugh a lot. But another friend comes with his father, who's a doctor. His dad keeps asking me about my chemo and the vomiting. I know he means well, but to tell you the truth, I don't really want to talk about it."*

Daniel was starting to recognize which relationships worked for him, and I suggested he refrain from seeing those he didn't want to.[5] This is not always easy, and it can be helpful to ask someone else to serve as intermediary in situations like this.

Practice for Healthy Living

Keep away from those who focus only on the disease and insist on talking about what's not working well and what's going wrong. Keep away from anyone who might encourage you to think and act in ways you'd rather not.

Stay with those who are willing to change with you and adapt to your needs, as you seek healthier lifestyle choices.

Surround yourself by people who believe in you—who believe you are more than your physical body and can see the depth of your soul.

Spending more time in **the company of those who believe in a wider approach to the health-disease process** supports your efforts to stimulate your immune system.

I received a call from Esther's husband, wanting medical advice. Esther had been admitted to the Emergency Room at the hospital, short of breath. She was diagnosed with a mesothelioma, a tumor that affects the pleura or membrane covering the lungs. He insisted on having our first appointment without her present. When we met, he was accompanied by his brother and one of their sons. The men were anxious to know what they could do for her and wanted to connect with a specialist in the US.

I talked with them for a long time. After describing the holistic viewpoint on cancer, I told them that it was important to include Esther in future meetings, explaining that integrative oncology means the "patient" participates fully and takes responsibility for all efforts, decisions, and discipline.

The word *patient* is related to patience, which we think means inactivity—that a patient needs to behave himself, exercise little curiosity, ask few questions, and request almost no explanations. This approach conditions us toward passivity, which is why I prefer the term *person seeking advice.* I call each person seeking advice by name, recognizing him or her as a whole person.

I explained why it was essential for Esther to take an active role in her own recovery process. My role, I said, is to offer tools that can make her stronger and be more empowered to cope with *her symptoms, treatment, and whatever else life brings.*

Responsibility (response-ability) is crucial. The person seeking advice sets aside passivity and looks for answers from the doctor and any other resources that can help bring about a fuller understanding of the disease and a healthier lifestyle.

Many people make unhealthy lifestyle choices, e.g., smoking, excessive drinking, staying in toxic relationships. Then when they get sick, they seek medical advice as though it's the doctor who is primarily responsible for their health. It'd be like thinking your mechanic is responsible for your car even if you forget to put water in the radiator or change the oil. The mechanic can help with major repairs, but you're in charge of keeping the car in good condition. In the same way, responsibility for how you live and for your own happiness depends on you, and you can't give that responsibility to others.

Ana Paula, a forty-three-year-old who worked at a digital marketing company, had been diagnosed with breast cancer with metastasis to the brain. She came to me after consulting with four other oncologists and feeling unsatisfied with each of them. I sensed she had consumerist skills and tendencies, and sure enough, after receiving her diagnosis, she searched the web assiduously for anticancer supplements and herbs. She opened a small suitcase and showed me the many products she was taking: vitamins from the US, noni from Peru, graviola from Brazil, and much, much more. She indicated that she drank alcohol and smoked pot daily and had experimented with psychedelics.

I encouraged Ana Paula to be more objective and critical about what she reads on the web, especially in relation to supposed "anticancer" products. To give her an example, I asked, "When you buy a weightloss product, do you really believe you're going to lose all the pounds they promise?" Some manufacturers who sell "anticancer" products know how desperate people with cancer are and how they search for a miracle cure, and many take advantage of this. We're living in an age that allows people to have lots of information, but discernment is necessary. It's important to review possible interactions between medicines and over-the-counter products with a doctor or pharmacist. Over-the-counter products don't require comprehensive studies, and in most cases, interactions with other compounds aren't even analyzed. A salesman's job is to sell, not necessarily to ensure good health.

Ana Paula also suffered from diabetes, and her kidneys were challenged, so I recommended she stop taking noni because the preparation included large amounts of sugar and potassium, both taxing on the kidneys. I also warned her about the effects of daily alcohol and marijuana and continued speaking about this in our next session.

Luz was thirty-one and had two small children when she came to see me for medical advice. She had traveled twelve hours, from Neuquén, a province in Patagonia about 700 miles southwest of Buenos Aires. After a year of feeling tired, dizzy, and nauseous, she found that a magnetic resonance imaging

(MRI) showed a pineal tumor. The pineal gland is in the center of the brain and is involved in the secretion of certain hormones that, among other functions, regulate the sleep cycle.

It was a strange tumor, and it wasn't possible to determine when it had appeared. She visited several neuro-oncologists and received very different recommendations. They didn't agree on the best treatment or on the urgency to begin treatment. Surgery offered the best possible cure but had many possible long-term complications and consequences.

She was inclined to wait before undergoing a surgery, but most of the doctors she'd seen were unable to understand her position. "I'm not ready for surgery now," she told me. "What if, after surgery, I'm no longer able to speak or to hug my children? I want to be sure that I am leaving them rich experiences and education for the rest of their lives, so they can remember me in the best way possible."

For Luz, it was important to prepare herself to face surgery. Considering the uncertainty surrounding her case and the possibility that the tumor had been growing slowly for many years, I felt at ease supporting her on her proposal. She was taking responsibility and was committed to continuing periodic visits with her local doctor to detect quickly any changes that might arise. I suggested she find a therapist in Neuquén who could teach her relaxation, visualization, and bodywork techniques to help her connect with her inner self. In the meantime, we would stay in touch through email and Skype.

I told Luz that the old paradigm places the doctor in a position of supreme authority, where the patient only has to follow orders and ingest prescriptions. In the integrative approach, the person seeking advice assumes an active role, fully participating in her own recovery. The doctor, obviously, is specialized in medical treatments and knows which surgery is best and which medicines the most appropriate for the issue at hand. But the person seeking advice needs to understand what is going on and to take part in deciding what's best for her through participating in the search for the origins of the disease. This complementary information is critical, since the doctor can never fully get it, even with knowledge, empathy, examinations, lab analyses, and sophisticated studies.

The doctor benefits when patients are **proactive.** His or her role, then, is to help the person seeking advice **find a new balance.** The body of the person who is unwell is not merely a container carrying a disease inside. He or she is a person with emotions, thoughts, family history, and relationships that seem to be out of balance.

This means **re-envisioning the relationship between the doctor and healthcare team and the patient seeking advice.** Besides offering optimal medical care, the healthcare team must proactively help the person recover her or his balance. My experience has taught me to respect the reason each person believes is the cause of her or his disease or what is needed for recovery. My role, then, is one of guidance and counseling.

Health is not owned by doctors or the healthcare system. We can do a lot for ourselves to get better. In fact, we cannot grant this power to anyone else. We have the right (and responsibility, I'd say) to live healthier and happier lives and to seek help when we are out of balance. "You are seriously ill, and you can do something about it," I heard Carl Simonton, a pioneer in mind-body medicine,[6] say to people suffering with cancer.[7]

On a Skype call, Luz told me the steps she was taking. She'd found a well-trained and experienced psychologist, who worked with her using mind-body techniques. And while she was working to strengthen herself, she enjoyed time with her children and her husband. She was able to tell them in her own words the kind of surgery she needed, and she was able to address their fears and concerns and to cheer them up. Whatever happened, she told them, she would always love them.

Then one day I received an email from her. "Laura, I'm ready. In two weeks, I'll return to Buenos Aires for surgery." Six months had gone by. Now she felt ready to face surgery and the consequences it could bring.

Luz's surgery was successful, and the doctors were amazed at her quick recovery. Within a few days, she was walking, and she returned to Neuquén and her family. She recovered fully, with no complications. She had been able to forge her own healing path, self-designed as she consulted different specialists and, at the same time, listened to the needs of her body and her soul.

Healing emerges from a vision of wholeness, contemplating your wholeness as a human being.

Healing means "recovering integral health," and health is bio-psycho-social-spiritual wellness.

Thus, **healing is restoring our bio-psycho- social-spiritual wellness.**

Take-Home Message

We human beings are a complex and dynamic system.

Some key points to bear in mind when entering the healing path:

- Move stagnant and blocked energies.
- Focus daily on pleasant activities.
- Seek help. Know your healing limits.
- Surround yourself with those who believe in a comprehensive vision of the health-disease process.

An integrative approach to wellness implies:

- You are proactive, coming for medical advice. You commit to entering a healing path.
- Doctors are guides and experienced counselors.

Implicit in healing is a vision of wholeness. To heal is to restore your bio-psycho-social-spiritual wellness.

Chapter 5

ENERGIZE YOUR BODY!

> *I celebrate myself, and sing myself,*
> *And what I assume you shall assume,*
> *For every atom belonging to me as good belongs to you....*
> *Nature without check with original energy.*
> —WALT WHITMAN

In chapter 3, "Why Do We Get Sick?" we saw that illness occurs when the immune system and PNIE network are not in balance. In this chapter, we'll focus on the ability each of us has for self-healing.

Self-Healing Means Taking Care of Ourselves.

Heal is a synonym of *cure*, from Latin *curare*,[1] which means *take care of.*

When we take care of ourselves, we pave the way for self-healing, our *salutogenic* potential,[2] i.e., the ability to promote our own health. *Salutogenesis* is the opposite of *pathogenesis,* which is the emphasis of modern medicine, focusing on the factors that cause disease. With this approach, mainstream medicine has lost the integral perspective of the human being and our potential for self-healing. In addition to asking why we get sick, integrative medicine asks what we can do to stay healthy or become healthy again. Primary factors that promote health and well-being include eating nutritional foods mindfully, engaging in regular physical activity, and getting enough sleep.

The World Health Organization[3] concludes that modifying or avoiding key risk factors can significantly reduce the burden of cancer. These risk factors include:

- tobacco use, including cigarettes and smokeless tobacco
- being overweight or obese
- unhealthy diet with low fruit and vegetable intake
- lack of physical activity
- alcohol use
- sexually transmitted human papillomavirus (HPV) infection
- hepatitis or other carcinogenic infections
- ionizing and ultraviolet radiation
- urban air pollution
- indoor smoke from household use of solid fuels[4]

In addition to these factors, the way we face everyday life and the way we relate to others significantly influence our health. Chapter 7, "The Treasure Hunt," and chapter 9, "Tuning Up," will address these influences.

We know that chronic stress can produce an imbalance and a loss of energy. When a system fails, there's little energy left to reorganize, transform, or promote self-healing. That's why it's so important—from the very beginning—to take all necessary steps to energize the body, to harness energy, and to help it circulate well to supply our whole body-mind-spirit.

Exercising, eating, and sleeping give us energy, stimulate our immune system, and promote health. What kinds of exercise are recommended? What is a healthy diet? What does sleeping well mean?

Julieta, a thirty-eight-year-old sports teacher, came to me after a mammogram showed a lesion in one breast and a biopsy confirmed that it was a malignant tumor. Although she exercised regularly, both indoors and out, she felt pressured by her work as a teacher and, due to financial concerns, had to hold a second job to support herself. She had been in a relationship, but when she came to see me, she was living alone. Besides work-related stress, disappointments in relationships had made her anxious.

Practice for Healthy Living

Notice how you fill your tank.

Ingesting healthy food and drink is one way. But sometimes when we're feeling exhausted, physically and mentally, eating something or drinking coffee doesn't seem to help.

There are other ways to reenergize your system:

Getting enough sleep.

Breathing consciously.

Exercising.

Calming your mind through meditation or other practices that clear the mind.

Devoting time to something you love.

Meeting with people you enjoy, and having a good time.

Connecting with what you care about most in life.

We feel love when we flow with the energy we generate and receive.

"Laura, I'm frightened," she told me. "While I wait for the operation, the cancer keeps growing. Is there anything I can do to help my body heal?"

Considering that illness shows a systemic imbalance and that Julieta would undergo a highly invasive treatment, we talked about how she might prepare herself to be in the best shape possible for the surgery. I suggested she imagine how she would train for a long-distance race. She'd have to maintain a balanced diet, constantly eliminating toxins, and get enough rest to be strong.

I added that a healthy diet, staying hydrated, eliminating toxins, exercising, and getting enough rest are not just for facing surgery. We need this much self-care every day, and especially when we're facing a systemic imbalance and need to activate the body's wisdom to strengthen our immune system, awaken our power of self-healing, and be ready to face the needed treatments.

Stress and the contingencies of life can distance us from healthy habits. Ancient healing systems like Ayurveda propose four factors for maintaining health: exercise, nutrition, healthy routines, and mental harmony. We'll look into the first three factors here, and the fourth, mental harmony, in chapter 9, "Tuning Up."

Good daily habits are critical. They encourage the expression of genes that help the immune system work properly and depress the activity of those that predispose us to illnesses, including cancer. Unhealthy habits increase the likelihood of becoming ill or developing a chronic disease. **How we live is important.**

Avoiding tobacco use, maintaining a healthy weight, exercising, and eating a balanced diet can reduce the risk of developing cancer significantly. **Up to 60 percent of cancers can be prevented with healthy habits. Furthermore, once cancer is diagnosed, healthy habits can reduce the disease's progression.** A study involving men with low-grade prostate cancer who chose not to undergo surgery, hormonal therapy, or radiation showed that nutrition and exercise can positively impact a diagnosed cancer. The men in this study changed their lifestyles, eating healthily, exercising moderately, managing stress, and attending support groups. In three months, these lifestyle changes slowed the progress of the disease, allowing some of the men to postpone or cancel surgery or radiation.

Healthy lifestyle changes not only reduced cancer markers, but also positively impacted the expression of genes. Cancer-fighting genes were turned on, while those that lead to cancer development were turned off.[5] Other studies showed how curcumin (a turmeric-based supplement)[6] or resveratrol (found in grapes, red wine, dark chocolate, and blueberries; a substance produced by certain plants in response to injury or when the plant is under attack by pathogens)[7] can selectively activate or deactivate gene expression. In this way, they can inhibit cancer spread or maximize chemotherapy's effects.

Julieta asked, *"Are you saying that if I go on a strict diet and continue exercising, I can be cured of my cancer?"*

I explained that it's not as simple as that. Some authors say this, but I don't believe we function in such a linear way. Once our system is out of balance, setting it right can be difficult. Although the research I cited for Julieta does show that in some cases of early prostate cancer, treatment can be postponed, we cannot expect the same results for all patients with prostate or any type or stage of cancer. It does, however, confirm that diet and exercise do affect cancer.

There may be cases in which cancer regresses or disappears when you eat more healthfully, but that's not the same as saying a good diet is a cure for cancer. In many cases, people undergo other changes in their lifestyle as well. Each case is unique. There isn't a single healing formula for all people and all cases.

A healthy diet is necessary, but not sufficient. Self-treatment with only diet misses the opportunity of a cure that might require a combination of therapies,—conventional ones and those focused on strengthening the immune system, including diet, exercise, humor, and stress management.

One of these exceptional cases is that of Dr. David Servan-Schreiber,[8] who, following a drastic change in lifestyle, lived almost twenty years without his brain cancer recurring. In his last book, *Anticancer: A New Way of Life,*[9] a *New York Times* best seller that's been translated into thirty-five languages, he writes about his diagnosis at age thirty-one and the treatment program he put together to heal himself beyond his surgery, chemo, and radiation. He adopted a healthy diet, exercised, practiced meditation, and began other mind-body therapies to deal with stress, difficult emotions, and relationships and to connect what made him happy. His **healthy diet** was part of an integrative treatment that included **exercise** and **stress management. These are important pillars of any cancer recovery program.**

Habits are ways we act, think, wish, or feel repeatedly, often unconsciously, sometimes compulsively. Habits can be difficult to break because they're imprinted on our neural circuitry, some of them since childhood.[10] When we walk the same path over and over, a groove is formed and we tend to fall into the same patterned movement if we don't make an arduous effort to do something different. To alter the groove, we need first to become aware of it. Only then can we change it and create a new habit and a new path. For example, if we become aware that we always choose red meat for dinner, we see that we could just as easily choose chicken or fish and create a healthier habit. Neuroscience teaches *plasticity,* that our brains are malleable and shapeable and can form new pathways. Neural plasticity, also called neuroplasticity or synaptic plasticity, is the brain's capacity to form new nerve pathways *throughout our life* in response to new information, sensory stimulation, development, dysfunction, or damage. Neuroplasticity, the "renewal of cerebral wiring," allows us to rewire the way we sense and respond to the world.

To me, habits are within the software of our energetic system, like an energetic 3D cobweb that runs through us and goes beyond our physical boundaries.

Replacing unhealthy habits with healthy ones is an important effort we can make toward reestablishing balance. To change a habit, first become aware of it; second, decide to change; third, provide conditions that increase the likelihood of change; fourth, identify new ways to act; and finally, try them out. Expect to fail or relapse sometimes, but continue to focus on the healthy habit you want.

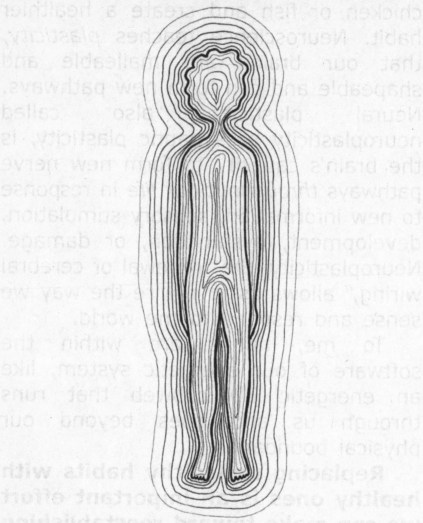

Our energetic system.

Each of our habits is a pattern within a large energetic network that overlays body and mind. **To change a habit,** instructing the brain is not enough; **the body must also be involved.** Practicing yoga or some other conscious movement, we begin to loosen the grip of these energetic patterns, increase the network's flexibility, and in the process become conscious of some habits. Doing this allows us to undo habits that are no longer useful and search for and test-drive healthier patterns. A change in an embodied habit brings forth new possibilities and makes changing other habits, like diet or sleep patterns, easier.

The first step is to **become aware.** Then, focusing on the body, ask yourself, Do I feel well in my body? Am I flexible? Is my weight healthy? Is what I eat health-affirming? Do I feel rested when I wake up? If you're uncertain about any of these, look at it and see if you're ready to make changes that can help you feel better.

An important first step toward a healthier life is to **make a reasonable and acceptable commitment.** It can help to put it in writing and link it to an intention, such as, "Today I will pay more attention to what I eat, go for walks, and take short breaks throughout the day to encourage my recovery."

Changing a habit means forming a new neural pathway. If we keep spending time in the same places with the same people acting the same way, it's difficult to change a habit. This is certainly the case for smokers who have rituals like going to a café and smoking or stepping outside with colleagues during breaks at work to smoke and chat together. If a smoker decides to stop smoking and continues the same rituals, it will be difficult if not impossible to stop. Just as a seed needs favorable conditions to germinate, we need **favorable conditions to enact the changes we want and to make them last.**

Practice for Healthy Living

What are you ready to commit to? Write it on a piece of paper and put it in a visible place as a daily reminder. It helps to make a commitment and work diligently to stick to it.

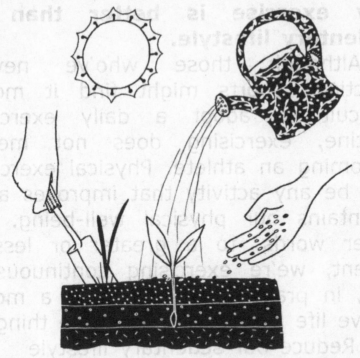

The need to create favorable conditions.

Let us now review healthy habits we might adopt with regard to exercise, diet, and sleep. Dealing with stress, learning to live with uncertainty, and seeing how we relate to others also strongly affect our health, and we'll analyze these in chapter 9, "Tuning Up."

Physical Exercise

Although each of us has our own preferences, abilities, and limitations,

any exercise is better than a sedentary lifestyle.

Although those who've never practiced sports might find it more difficult to adopt a daily exercise routine, exercising does not mean becoming an athlete. Physical exercise can be any activity that improves and maintains our physical well-being. In other words, to a greater or lesser extent, we're exercising continuously. But, in practice, we can lead a more active life by focusing on three things:

- Reduce our sedentary lifestyle
- Assume a more active attitude in everyday life
- Devote time regularly to physical activity[11]

Physique

The word **physique** comes from the Greek *physikós*, which means "related to nature."

Physical exercise connects our body with our environment.

Regardless of our activity level, the time we spend sitting or lying down, using the computer, or watching TV affects our health. The time we spend sitting increases the risk of obesity, Type 2 diabetes, some types of cancer, and the risk of dying at an earlier age. Therefore, it's important to **limit our sedentary time. Identify which daily activities are sedentary** and find ways to modify them. For example, when working at the computer, stand up every fifteen minutes and take a few steps. At the office, walk to your colleague's workstation rather than phoning him or sending an email.

Choose physical activity when you can. Climb the stairs instead of using the elevator, walk, and use public transportation or ride a bike instead of driving. Get off the train or bus one stop before your destination and complete the trip on foot. Take a break during work to go for a short walk. Counting the number of steps you take daily with a pedometer or a smartphone app can help you become aware and increase your walking.

Practice for Healthy Living

In the same way that you spend time eating and sleeping, spend time exercising every day.

In addition to these kinds of changes throughout the day, set aside time to **exercise regularly.**

The American Cancer Society recommends engaging in at least **two-and-a-half hours of moderately intense activity or an hour and fifteen minutes of vigorously intense activity (or an equivalent combination) each week, preferably spread throughout the week.** Moderately intense activities are "those that require effort equivalent to that of a brisk walk." Vigorously intense activities "generally engage large muscle groups and cause a noticeable increase in heart rate, breathing depth and frequency, and sweating."[12]

The following are examples of moderate and vigorous-intensity activities:[13]

	MODERATE-INTEN-SITY	VIGOROUS-INTEN-SITY
Recreational exercises and activities	Walking briskly, dancing, cycling, ice or roller skating, horseback riding, canoeing, practicing yoga	Jogging or running, cycling quickly, weight training, aerobic dancing, martial arts, jumping rope, swimming.
Sports	Volleyball, golf, baseball, tennis doubles, downhill skiing.	Soccer, field or ice hockey, tennis singles, basketball, cross-country skiing.
Home activities	Mowing the lawn and general lawn and garden maintenance.	Digging, carrying and hauling, masonry and carpentry.
Activities at the workplace	Walking and lifting as part of farming, auto or machine repair.	Heavy manual labor related to forestry and construction.

Current Research

Some experts say that two-and-a-half hours of moderate physical activity a week is too ambitious. They suggest that sedentary individuals can focus on small increases in physical activity each day and that those already physically active who don't have extra time can combine activities of varied intensity that fit into their schedules.[14]

High-intensity interval training (HIT) alternates short bursts of vigorous exercise, such as sprinting the way our ancestors must have run when they went hunting, with periods of moderate activity or rest. HIT reaches a high level of cardiovascular demand more quickly and efficiently than most other kinds of intense exercise. The results of HIT are pretty much the opposite of a sedentary life. Researchers are exploring whether some of HIT's positive effects, e.g., the reduction of fasting insulin, abdominal fat, and inflammation, might also reduce the risk of cancer.[15]

Abdominal fat has been associated with increased risk of colorectal cancer and, down the road, of pancreatic, endometrial, and breast cancer in postmenopausal women. Adipose tissue, or fat, particularly abdominal adipose tissue, produces pro-inflammatory cytokines such as the tumor necrosis factor alpha

(TNF-alpha) or interleukin-1 (IL-1). Cytokines, small proteins that are important in cell signaling, can also cause cell death. They promote metabolic syndrome, which raises the risk of heart disease, stroke, cancer, and diabetes. Muscles can be considered endocrine organs, since they communicate with other organs through the secretion of cytokines called myokines. These are different from those secreted by the adipose tissue, since myokines produce anti-inflammatory effects, blocking the development of metabolic syndrome, increasing insulin sensitivity, and increasing of intramuscular glucose use. HIT eliminates adipose tissue and inhibits the secretion of pro-inflammatory cytokines, while stimulating muscles to secrete myokines. HIT is an excellent regimen for those whose schedules don't allow for long periods of physical activity.

Why wait till tomorrow? You can start today.

Walking is an excellent exercise, and it only takes a pair of walking shoes and choosing a time of day. Unless you have a physical impairment, you can do it. To create favorable conditions, invite a relative or friend to join you at a fixed day and time. You'll encourage each other, and you'll both benefit.

People exercise to reduce weight, improve cardiovascular functioning, maintain muscle tone, and look fit. Exercise provides energy and encourages living actively by delivering nutrients and oxygen to the tissues.[16] It also improves the quality of sleep. High-intensity exercise boosts the production of endorphins, which make us feel happy, even euphoric, increasing our self-esteem and self-confidence[17] and helping people overcome depression.[18] In addition to these benefits, exercise stimulates the immune system, improves health,[19] extends longevity, and reduces the risk of dying from some types of cancer.

Exercise also has positive effects on the brain and its functions. It reduces anxiety and helps us cope with stressors by increasing norepinephrine or noradrenaline levels. Norepinephrine is a neurotransmitter that modulates the stress response. Half of it is produced in the *locus coeruleus*, a region of the brain that connects the areas involved in emotions and stress. Some antidepressants increase the brain levels of norepinephrine. Some psychologists believe that exercise increases our capacity to respond to stressors, since it enhances communication among the musculoskeletal, cardiovascular, endocrine, and autonomic nervous systems. The more sedentary we are, the less efficient our body is in responding to stressors.

Practice for Healthy Living

Exercise at least thirty minutes a day.

Exercise can help improve your mood, reduce stress, and maintain mental stability. Those who exercise find it easier to change unhealthy habits.

Physical activity improves memory and learning, counteracting the cognitive decline that begins at age forty-five and affects thinking, reasoning, learning, and memory. Exercise, especially for those between twenty-five and forty-five, increases the neurotransmitters that prevent hippocampus deterioration, involved in memory and learning.[20] Exercise also helps us control addictions, e.g., to sweets or food in general. With exercise, the brain releases dopamine, the pleasure hormone, as a response to exercise, sex, alcohol, drugs, food, or other pleasurable experiences. When we produce dopamine through, e.g., exercise, we'll lessen its release through other stimuli, for example, eating. And when we exercise, we encourage others to do the same.

Be creative in establishing an exercise routine that works for you. Walking is a great activity, but it can be difficult to find the time to walk several times a week. When you're sick, people want to help, but they don't know what you need. Ask them to **walk with** you every week at a fixed time. Finding one person for one day each week and someone else for another day will make it easier to establish a walking routine.

Other ways to encourage an exercise routine include listening to music you love while you're on a bike or a walking machine, joining a sports team in your neighborhood, exercising instead of eating out, going for a walk in the park, or visiting a new neighborhood. You can dance with a partner or friends or organize a dance party at home. Or just select a playlist that encourages you to dance a while every day. Plan walking tours, biking, or outdoor activities on holidays instead of trips that involve only driving.

Those who are inactive or just beginning a physical regimen can begin slowly and gradually and then add more. Men over forty, women over fifty, and those with a chronic disease or cardiovascular risk factors should consult their physician before beginning any program of physical activity.

What Is Your Relationship with Your Body?

Do you say, I have a body? If so, who is this *I* who has a body?

Do you say, I am a body? If so, does "body" include mind and soul?

These questions have engaged philosophers throughout time.

In the Biblical tradition, man consists of body and soul. All human experiences—not only those clearly involving the body such as eating, dancing, and sleeping, but also those considered intangible, like thinking, remembering, and loving—are lived in the body.

In contrast, Plato held the dualistic view that body and soul are separate realities. The body is the ship and the soul is the captain who guides it. Descartes[21] affirmed this Platonic idea and, based on Newtonian mechanics,[22] described the human body as a machine. The soul, which he called *consciousness,* although linked to the body, is separate from it.

Since Descartes, science has been studying the body and religions have been studying the soul. This dualistic worldview has characterized several centuries of Western history and led to a devaluation of the body to the point of considering sexuality a sin.[23]

We live in a **reductionist paradigm** in which everything can be divided into parts, analyzed, and then reassembled. The human being does not operate that way. We are not machines; we cannot divide ourselves and reassemble the pieces afterward.

For the last few decades, we have been revaluing the spiritual dimension amid an increasing interest in the human being as a whole, and a **holistic paradigm** is reappearing. We are a whole person, with body, mind, heart, and spirit.[24]

The intention is not only to exercise but also to create a better relationship with your body. We live in a society that believes that mind and body are separate, as though mind is the control tower and body the incoming aircraft, or a possession we take around with us.

How many times do we try to do more than our body can, yet our mind keeps making demands, ignoring the body's signals, such as headaches, fatigue, and pain? We take a painkiller and keep going until something more serious overcomes us, like flu or pneumonia. **The body whispers, then it talks, and then it shouts that something is out of order.**

There are many kinds of conscious bodywork,[25] including yoga, breathwork, qigong, and taiji, that help us create a different kind of relationship with our body. Through these practices, we begin to hear what the body is teaching us, and we can apply this knowledge to other areas of our life. For example, practicing yoga, we learn to recognize our limits and discover that our ability and capacity varies from day to day and that we're more flexible in certain situations than others.

Our body shapes itself according to the experiences we have and the ways we respond to them. We build up shields to protect us from painful or frightening situations. When we are ready for a healing journey, practices like bioenergetics can help us undo these protections. There are many techniques that focus on processing trauma in our body.[26]

The body retains its memory. Once we've learned to ride a bicycle, as soon as we get on one, even after many years, our body remembers what to do. Memory is not only stored in the brain. We know the hippocampus and the frontal cortex play important roles regarding memory, but scientists have not been able to locate a memory reservoir. Perhaps it's stored as an imprint in the brain-body complex.

Many holistic practitioners posit that our bodies store emotional memories. Some use the image of a cyst, saying that traumatic energies are enclosed in cysts, in the way the body encloses bacteria in an abscess. When someone is unable to process a traumatic experience in real time, that emotional energy might get buried, or encysted, in the body to be metabolized later. Some people describe these kinds of experiences using words like, "I felt the disease enter my body."

Have you ever seen someone experience a Eureka moment and burst into laughter during a yoga practice or a peak sports event? It might be the release of frustration, confusion, distress, pain, fear, or loss, exiting from the depths of our being, freeing us from something we've held for a long time. Releasing feelings that have until now been intolerable can quicken our gait, open our mind, and bring us to a state of bliss.

There are massage therapists, acupuncturists, chiropractors, and other conscious bodyworkers who can, at times, access our stored memories and help us release them. Being in certain bodily positions or making certain movements while our attention is focused within, images, memories, or feelings might arise that yield *insight*, unlocking what has been stored within.

Can any physical exercise be conscious bodywork? It depends on your mind, your approach, your attitude. If you watch TV while walking on a treadmill, your attention is outside. In yoga, you stay with your breath and how you feel. That is conscious bodywork.

Bioenergetics works with the tensions that suppress our feelings. Over time, the body forms more and more rigid structures, such as contractures, the shortening of muscles, tendons, or other tissues, affecting our ability to move with ease, our breathing patterns, and leading us to repeat certain movements. Bioenergetics helps us break these energetic patterns and release knots, giving us the possibility of contacting parts of our body that have been trapped.[28] In the same way that the body can open itself and expose hidden areas, we too can allow repressed feelings to come forth.

Let Your Body Drive

The French car maker Peugeot promoted one of its models with the slogan, "Let your body drive."[27]

I heard it as an invitation to stop living in our heads and **recognize our body's wisdom.**

The understanding that emotions are stored in the body is recognized by most body therapists but is not well accepted among scientists, because it can't be easily replicated within a controlled environment. Emotional release occurs spontaneously in each person and cannot be reproduced on request for study or evaluation.

When certain parts of the body are stimulated during exercise or bodywork, specific areas of the brain associated with emotional processing are affected. The limbic system, which is the center of emotions, is anatomically related to the brainstem, which controls breathing and cardiac rhythm, both of which are stimulated during physical exercise. By activating the limbic system, the center of emotions in the brain, exercise allows emotional memories to be accessed and processed.

Emotional release can be a pleasant experience. Oftentimes before the release, people feel like a "heavy backpack, difficult to carry" and after the experience, they feel lighter and in many cases, symptoms disappear. Freed from the burden, we find the strength and courage to change the course of our lives.

Nutrition

Let food be thy medicine,
and medicine be thy food.

—HIPPOCRATES

Antonio, a fifty-eight-year-old businessman, came to see me after he'd had surgery for colon cancer. He had read that an unhealthy diet and excessive weight could cause cancer. "Doctor," he said, "Can you recommend a weightloss diet?" When I asked him to tell me his basic diet, he talked about Sunday barbecues, breaded steaks on Tuesdays with friends, salami as an appetizer, and more. It was clear he was eating too much red meat.

I explained to Antonio that eating a healthy diet is essential for keeping the body well, that we need to **take responsibility for the way we eat.** A sedentary lifestyle combined with stress and an unhealthy diet, including animal fat, sugar, and processed food, contribute to the body's production of substances that cause chronic inflammation. Inflammation is the body's response to a wound or to protect us from infection, and normally it disappears after accomplishing its goal. An excessive or extended inflammatory reaction increases our susceptibility to cardiovascular disease, diabetes, and even cancer.

How can we block inflammation? Excessive body fat, consumption of too many calories, and low activity levels increase the risk of many types of cancer—breast (in postmenopausal women), colon and rectal, endometrial, esophageal, kidney, pancreatic, gallbladder, liver, non-Hodgkin lymphoma, multiple myeloma, uterine, cervical, ovarian, and prostate. Regular exercise, anti-stress practices,[29] and particularly a healthy diet can reduce many kinds of cancer and increase the chances of recovery in those diagnosed with cancer.

Antonio tried to negotiate. *"I've made up my mind and will do whatever's necessary to stop cancer from returning, but Doctor, are you going to forbid me Sunday barbecues? What if I play a round of golf Sunday mornings?"*

Unfortunately, **no exercise of any kind or in any amount can** produce enough anti-inflammatory substances to **offset the inflammation produced by an unhealthy diet.** The best place to start is to follow a healthy, anti-inflammatory diet.

Practice for Healthy Living

Let the shopping list be your recipe.

Let the kitchen be your drugstore.

Let food be your medicine.

Although **there is no single formula for a healthy diet** as each of us has different needs and tastes, an anti-inflammatory diet needs to be based on more vegetables and fewer animal products. Diet also needs to take into account the specific needs of each stage of surgery and recovery, chemotherapy (see Neutropenic Diet), and periods of diarrhea or constipation.

A diet that is beneficial for one person might not be for someone else, but **there are some basic recommendations for everyone.** Research on what is a healthy diet is continuously evolving. There are products not included in these recommendations that can be beneficial but to date don't have enough medical evidence of anticancer effectiveness. The fact that they have not been sufficiently tested doesn't mean they're not effective. Since this knowledge base is alive and continuously being updated, it's advisable to periodically review reliable sources devoted to this issue and update your understanding of what is the healthiest diet for you.

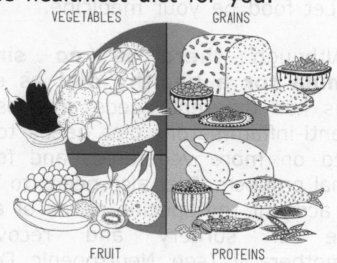

Healthy diet.

Basic Recommendations for a Healthy Diet

Maintain a healthy weight, calculated as body mass index (BMI), which factors in your height and weight. Generally, the higher the BMI, the more body fat you have, although there are exceptions, and it can vary between men and women.

To calculate BMI, Google "BMI," and an interactive chart will appear.

- **BMI of 18.5 to 25** is considered normal, or healthy.
- **25 to 30** is considered overweight.
- **30 or higher** indicates obesity.

Eat little red meat (a pound or less per week) or processed meat (cold cuts) and choose white meats (organic free-range chicken, wild-caught fish (not farm-raised). When eating red meat, choose cuts without fat and eat small portions.

Reduce fat intake. Replace fried foods with meals prepared using other cooking methods, such as steaming or roasting. When using fats, reduce animal fats (such as meat and dairy products, or use skim versions), and replace them with vegetable fats. Among vegetable oils, avoid trans fats, such as margarine or other hydrogenated oils found in processed foods, such as biscuits, fast foods, fried and pastry products (see appendix 1, "Nutrition").Trans fatty acids or trans fats are a type of unsaturated fat produced during the hydrogenation process to solidify them so they will display well and have a longer shelf life. Trans fats as well as omega-6 fatty acids are pro-inflammatory. They can be particularly dangerous for the heart and are associated with a higher risk of developing some kinds of cancer. Oils rich in omega-3, like flaxseed and fish oils, are anti-inflammatory. Among vegetable oils, one of the best choices is extra virgin olive oil. Olive oil is a monounsaturated fat with vitamins A and E, magnesium, and a variety of heart-protective nutrients.

Eat two- and-a-half cups or five units of a variety of fruits and vegetables daily,[30] preferably raw (see Neutropenic Diet). The more vegetables, the better. And whenever possible if it's within your budget, choose organic fruits and vegetables.[31] It's recommended not to eat more than two pieces of fruit per day, though, to avoid excessive sugar intake. A fun way to consume vegetables and fruits is by making smoothies or juices that maintain the fiber. Extracts aren't recommended because they destroy the fiber and leave only a sugary liquid.

Fiber encourages a healthy gastrointestinal transit and can serve as a prebiotic to feed colon bacteria that help digestion, reduce inflammation, help absorb nutrients gradually and avoid sugar rushes, and reduce the risk of some types of cancer, especially colorectal cancer. Avoid certain fruits, such as grapefruit, while you are receiving chemotherapy: Grapefruit interferes with one of the cytochrome P enzymes—CYP3A, the substance in your body responsible for metabolizing chemotherapy drugs like docetaxel (which is used for breast, lung, and prostate cancers). It can make the drug more potent, thus more toxic.[32]

Replace white and refined flours with whole wheat flour, and replace

white rice with whole grain rice. Whole grain flours and rice keep the entire grain, including the bran, where healthy fibers and vitamins reside. During the refining process, the bran is discarded and the refined product consists mainly of complex sugars. Choose products such as breads, pasta, and cereals completely made out of whole or integral grains, instead of refined products.

Minimize consumption of foods that have large amounts of added sugars. Sugar increases calorie intake and may indirectly increase cancer risk.[34] White (refined) sugar, brown (unrefined) sugar, and honey produce similar effects. It's recommended that you reduce the consumption of sweetened foods such pastries, cakes, sugary cereals, ice cream, candy, jam and marmalade, soda, and energy drinks sweetened with sugar. If you want something sweet, eat fruit or dark chocolate with high cacao content and no added sugar. To sweeten, sugar can be replaced with stevia, which is extracted from the leaves of a plant native to South America. Lately it's being raised commercially as well. Intermittent fasting[35] is a way to overcome the addiction to sweets. Cutting down on sugar also calms the mind.

Neutropenic Diet

During chemotherapy treatment, on some days the immune system will weaken—when the absolute neutrophil count (ANC) is lower than 1,500 or 1,000, called *neutropenia*—and it's critical to maintain good hygiene. Neutropenia is an abnormally low level of neutrophils, a common type of white blood cell important to fighting off infections, particularly those caused by bacteria.

During this period, the risk of infection can be reduced by washing your hands with antibacterial soap and warm water several times a day, especially after using the toilet and before preparing food. The risk of infection can also be reduced by eating a *neutropenic* diet. For those who have had bone marrow transplants, nutrition restrictions need to be observed even more strictly.

A neutropenic diet consists of:

• avoiding raw foods or foods cooked rare, whether meat, fish, eggs, or tofu.

• avoiding foods that aren't fresh or safe, e.g., date expired, prepared in poor hygienic conditions, cooked food left out of the refrigerator for two or more hours, moldy cheeses such as brie, feta, or blue.

• avoiding moldy or unwashed fruits and vegetables. It isn't necessary to avoid raw fruits or vegetables since there is no evidence that they promote infection, but they must be very well washed before consuming.[33]

• avoiding raw vegetables in restaurants or places where you're not sure they were washed properly. Sprouts must always be cooked.

• avoiding unpasteurized honey or beverages, including fruit or vegetable juice, beer, and milk

• consuming high-quality proteins to rebuild white blood cells.

> • taking mineral and vitamin supplements if needed.

Read the Labels!

Bread made *with* whole wheat flour is not the same as bread made *of* whole wheat flour. The former uses white or refined flour and adds whole wheat flour. The latter is made completely out of whole wheat flour.

Limit consumption of milk and dairy products. Milk's fats, hormones, and calcium can produce harmful effects and increase the risk of some cancer types (see "Milk and Dairy Products" in the glossary in appendix 1, "Nutrition"). If you need to consume more calcium for bone health, eat leafy green vegetables (spinach, watercress and broccoli, parsley, basil), legumes, nuts, and seeds, such as sesame, and be certain to keep vitamin D levels adequate for efficient calcium absorption and metabolism.

Adequate levels of vitamin D can prevent some types of cancer and the recurrence of breast cancer. Low vitamin D levels may lead to increased risk of pancreatic, lung, ovarian, breast, prostate, and skin cancer. Research on menopausal women showed that cancer risk may be reduced 77 percent with serum vitamin D levels of at least 40 ng/ml.[36] Sunbathing (avoid peak hours) is the best source of active vitamin D. Vitamin D is also present in certain foods, such as fatty fish, eggs, avocado, and vitamin-fortified products like orange juice and fortified cereals. If necessary, take vitamin supplements. The dosage should be adjusted to your current vitamin D level.

Practice for Healthy Living

Vitamin D varies for each person according to sun exposure and nutrition. Ask your doctor to check the vitamin D level in your blood at least every six months.

To optimize your health, your level must be between 50 and 70 ng/ml. If your vitamin D level is lower than 40 ng/ml, you can take supplements.

Add antioxidants that inhibit free radicals—produced during metabolism or through contact with toxins, by pollution or infections—which are responsible for cellular degeneration (see "Antioxidants and Phytochemicals" in the glossary in appendix 1, "Nutrition"). In order to keep our cells healthy, it's important to add enough antioxidants to your diet, mainly fruits (especially citrus fruits such as oranges, and red fruits such as raspberries, strawberries, and blueberries), vegetables, green tea, and chocolate. Spices such as turmeric and fats containing omega-3 are also good sources. Cooking with garlic, onions, and ginger increases foods' antioxidant and anti-inflammatory properties.

Add foods that strengthen the immune system, such as yeast, garlic, onions, lemon, papaya, pumpkin, broccoli, Brussels sprouts, sauerkraut, legumes, fruits, vegetables in general, and water kefir. The latter is probiotic, as it provides live and active microorganisms that can help balance intestinal flora and strengthen the immune system.

Add foods that help to keep the detoxification organs—liver, kidneys, skin, and lungs—clean. The detox organs remove toxins from our body. Toxins may come from diet, air, medicines, or substances produced through chemical reactions of our body's metabolism. The main detoxification organs are the liver and the kidneys. We also remove toxins when we exhale and perspire. Kidneys work closely with the immune system. An unhealthy diet and chronic exposure to toxins, together with other factors that prevent adequate detoxification, such as chronic stress, increase an organism's acidity and overload the kidneys, especially when one doesn't consume the micronutrients of a healthy diet. Under such conditions, the kidneys slow down and reduce their effectiveness, and toxins that threaten the immune system accumulate. As a consequence, the body triggers a global inflammation that, when chronic, is detrimental to the organism.[37] Certain foods help remove toxins: onions, parsley, artichokes, beets, broccoli, chard, spinach, arugula, lemon, garlic, asparagus, blueberries, oats, tomatoes, endive, lettuce, eggplant, apples, red currants, green beans, and pineapple. You can also drink detox infusions, but consult an integrative physician before doing so to be sure to select one that's beneficial for your condition and in accord with other medicines and supplements you're taking.[38]

Take probiotics and prebiotics. *Probiotics* contain live microorganisms (*bifidobacterium* and *lactobacillus*), and when administered in adequate amounts, they confer health benefits.[39] Lactobacilli live mainly in the small intestine and are necessary for digestion. Bifidobacteria live in the large intestine and contribute to processing foods until they're eliminated. Many factors can destabilize gut flora—stress, poor nutrition, antibiotics, constipation, and chemicals including additives, preservatives, and dyes. This destabilization can create inflammatory conditions, immune system depression, variations in the digestion and absorption of nutrients, and constipation. Besides fighting bacteria and restoring gut flora balance and digestion, probiotics strengthen the protective and anti-infective activity of the mucous membrane, skin, and immune system. *Prebiotics* are nondigestible carbohydrates that stimulate probiotics' growth and activity. The intake of probiotics and prebiotics contributes to the balance of the gut flora. In this way, they not only improve nutrient absorption, but also reduce inflammatory conditions and strengthen the immune system. Some research suggests that probiotics could have a role in cancer prevention.[40] Since they contain live microorganisms, **probiotics must not be used in case of a very low or depressed immune system.** Probiotics are present in water kefir, miso, rice water, or milk. Prebiotics are present in umeboshi plums, artichokes, legumes, asparagus, garlic, onions, leeks, oats, whole grain cereals, and barley.[41] Probiotics can be consumed in medicine or functional foods,[42] such as yogurt or fermented milks. Be careful! Not all the benefits you read on the labels have been proven in scientific studies.

Add Japanese mushrooms like *shiitake* **or** *maitake*, which seem to be beneficial for health. Diabetic patients taking hypoglycemic medications or people under anticoagulant treatment must consult their physician before consuming maitake mushrooms, because they interfere with these medications and can produce severe side effects. (See more about these in appendix 2, "Frequently Asked Questions About Treatment.")

Choose natural foods over processed foods. Choose foods with fewer chemicals and additives. In addition to going through complex processing steps, processed foods often contain additives, artificial flavoring, and other chemical ingredients. Generally, foods made of natural ingredients that are mechanically processed (cut, cooked) are not included in this category. Additives are any substances added to foods and drinks that have no nutritional value in themselves. They are used in the food industry to enhance products' appearance by altering color, smell, taste, or texture; to prolong shelf life; or to reduce costs. The body recognizes these chemical substances as strange. Not only are they not nutritious, they can produce harmful effects and increase the risk of diseases such as cancer. Processed foods generally contain sugar, salt, and unhealthy fats to make them more attractive and addictive. Added sugars, salts, and fats can trigger the release of dopamine, stimulating the regions of the brain that are also activated by cocaine and other addictive drugs.[45] Eating processed foods, we ingest more calories and consume sugar, salt, and fats in excess, which is harmful to our health.

Practice for Healthy Living

Dr. Odile Fernández, a physician who had cancer and was able to reverse it by making significant lifestyle changes including a healthy diet, identifies ten foods as essential for combating cancer: turmeric, flaxseed, tomato, red fruit, black grapes and red wine, cauliflower and broccoli, olive oil, green tea, and citrus fruits.[43]

Include them in your shopping list.[44]

Limit salt consumption of processed foods and snacks (potato chips, peanuts, snack mix, etc.), which normally include large amounts of sodium chloride. Since salt increases appetite, it is included in many food-industry products, including sweets, to stimulate consumption. High consumption of sodium has been associated with increased blood pressure, which is a risk factor in the development of cardio- and cerebrovascular diseases. High consumption of salt is also associated with an increase in stomach cancer. Besides increasing obesity and hypertension, it can be harmful because of the chemicals used during the salt-refining process. It's preferable to consume unrefined salts, like sea salt or Himalayan pink salt, that often include trace amounts of beneficial nutrients.

Practice for Healthy Living

Pay attention to what you consume.

When you go food shopping, allow enough time to read the labels.

Pay special attention to the number of calories and quantities of sugar, salt, and fats, and try to consume foods that have less of these substances.

Avoid foods containing trans fats, artificial sweeteners (aspartame, saccharin), preservatives, colorants (many colorants beginning with E are toxic,[46] for example, E102, Tartrazine), or taste enhancers (monosodium glutamate, MSG, which provides the *umami* flavor and can damage the nervous system). The human tongue picks up five basic tastes: sweet, sour, salty, bitter, and umami. Umami (from Japanese, meaning "delicious taste") is one of the first flavors a newborn encounters. Umami is found in breast milk, as well as tomatoes, parmesan cheese, shiitake mushrooms, bonito flakes, soy sauce, cured meats, and kombu seaweed.[47]

Alkalize the body. It's been observed that cancer incidence is increasing as we generate more acidity in our everyday lives due to stress and the foods we eat. Although we know that tumors are more acidic, it hasn't been proven that cancer can be prevented or reduced by alkalizing our body. What is certain is that normal cells must be in a slightly alkaline environment to function precisely and adequately. Blood continuously regulates itself to guarantee correct cell activity, optimize metabolism, and avoid metabolic acidosis. If pH values ("potential of hydrogen," a numeric scale that specifies the acidity or basicity of a liquid) are below seven, it can result in a life-threatening coma. We must ingest from the food and minerals we eat sufficient alkalinity to neutralize blood acidity (see "Alkalize Your Diet" in the glossary in appendix 1, "Nutrition"). If the diet does not provide sufficient alkalinity, the body utilizes the minerals—calcium, magnesium, and potassium—in bones, joints, teeth, and nails, leading to the weakening of the bones and a propensity to osteopenia and osteoporosis.[48] We need to alkalize our body to support the proper functioning of normal cells, including those in the immune system.

The pH Change You're Familiar With

You're probably familiar with the effects of certain pH changes. Candidiasis, or vaginal yeast infection, is caused by a fungus. When the pH is healthy, candidiasis lives harmlessly in the vagina. But when the vagina's natural pH changes (e.g., due to tight clothes, hormonal changes, antibiotics, or scented soaps), the fungi multiply, resulting in an infection called vaginal mycosis.

To alkalinize our organism, we need to reduce acidity and increase alkalinity. Acidity can be reduced by managing stress (for example, practicing conscious breathing while meditating or in daily life to achieve a beneficial exchange of carbon dioxide and oxygen[49]) and improving our dietary habits, both what and how we eat. Eating quickly or while stressed can increase acidity. Eating slowly and chewing each bite more, our saliva alkalinizes the food. Dietary recommendations, as noted above, include eating fewer acidic foods, more alkaline ones, and ingesting the minerals needed to offset acidic excess. Many fruits, specifically lemons, and vegetables are excellent alkalinizers.[50]

Practice for Healthy Living

Alkalinize your organism and activate your kidneys.

Start your day by drinking lemon juice in a glass of water.

Hydrate—drink enough water. Two-thirds or more of our body is water; staying hydrated is essential for our well-being. We lose water through breathing, perspiring, urinating, and defecating, so we must continuously replace water to preserve our well-being. Many people feel tired, with less mental clarity, when they're not sufficiently hydrated. Research shows disturbances in mood and concentration and an increase of headaches in women who don't drink enough water after exercising.[51] Chronic dehydration is one of the main reasons the body tends to stress. The quality of our water is also important; drinking good water, we get some of the salts and minerals we need.

Is Water Healthy?

Water is treated chemically to remove bacteria and other harmful substances for it to be drinkable. If our drinking water has traces of lead, cadmium, or arsenic, these substances accumulate in the body and cause disease. Home filtration systems can purify tap water.

Contemporary researchers posit that water has memory and carries electromagnetic fluctuations determining its properties. Viktor Schauberger, known as the "water magician," studied subtle energies in nature and the importance of water in all natural processes. Wolfgang Ludwig explored the water frequency pattern and its "healing capacity." Johann Grander developed a method to modify the inner structure of water molecules to create "vitalized water." Masaru Emoto explored the effects of human consciousness on the molecular structure of water, and his work became known through the movie *What the Bleep Do We Know?*[52] Even though many of his studies are preliminary, some specific effects have already been proven. For example, seed germination and plant growth benefit when electromagnetic fields are applied to water. Human beings are also sensitive to electromagnetic fields. Research has shown astronauts suffer diseases such as osteoporosis after living in space, outside of magnetic fields.

If the water we drink is charged with negative electromagnetic frequencies, it could make us more susceptible to disease. On the other hand, water charged with healthy frequencies could favor healing and recovery. Diamantine and solar water energizing methods, e.g., are based in part on these postulates.

Italian physicist Giuliano Preparata[53] described how water is the physical basis of multicellular organization in complex organisms. Mae-Wan Ho, biochemist and geneticist, has spent decades investigating the properties of the quantum coherence of water. We can maintain a global cohesion of the whole organism if we maintain the state of coherence of the water we are composed of. She compared it to an orchestra or a jazz band; each musician has absolute freedom to improvise his or her own melody if the rhythm and pulse of the whole band is followed. The same happens within the organism: each cell has its autonomous activity and, thanks to the water's state of coherence that functions as an inner ocean, they all sound in unison.[54] Research is being developed about the quantum coherence of water that will provide more useful information in the near future.

Limit alcohol consumption to not more than two drinks per day for men and one per day for women. This translates to a bottle of beer (12 ounces), a restaurant-sized glass of wine (5 ounces), or 3 shot glasses (less than 2 ounces) of distilled liquor. Alcohol increases the risk of several types of cancer, including mouth, throat, esophageal, liver, and colon. What matters is the amount of *alcohol* consumed, not so much whether it's beer, wine, or hard liquor. When alcohol interacts with tobacco, it produces an exponential growth in the risk of mouth, larynx, and esophageal cancer. That's why it's also recommended to **avoid tobacco,** whether smoking or chewing, or breathing secondhand smoke. Cigarette smoke causes disease due to high oxidative stress—the production of more free radicals than the body can detoxify—caused by the release of reactive nitrogen and oxygen species, thus damaging cells. Smoking causes 30 percent or more of all cancer deaths. In addition to the dried tobacco leaves, ingredients are added for flavor. Due to the complex mixture of chemicals produced by the combustion of tobacco and its additives, tobacco smoke contains more than 7,000 chemical substances (benzene, cyanide, methane, ammoniac, etc.), including more than seventy known carcinogens. In addition, tobacco smoke contains poisonous gases, including tar, carbon monoxide, nitrogen oxides, and radioactive substances. One of the strongest chemicals found in tobacco smoke, nicotine, is addictive. Nicotine is what produces the effect people seek.[55]

Basic Recommendations for a Healthy Diet

Maintain a healthy weight.

Eat little red meat.

Reduce fat intake.

Eat two- and-a-half cups or five units of fruits and vegetables daily.

Replace white or refined flours with whole wheat flour, and white rice with whole grain rice.

Minimize your consumption of foods with high amounts of added sugars.

Limit milk and dairy-product consumption.

Keep vitamin D at proper levels.

Eat more antioxidant foods.

Eat more foods that strengthen the immune system.

Eat more foods that help keep detoxification organs—liver, kidneys, skin, and lungs—clean.

Take probiotics and prebiotics.

Include Japanese mushrooms like shiitake or maitake mushrooms.

Eat natural foods rather than chemically processed foods.

Limit salt consumption.

Alkalinize the organism.

Drink enough good-quality water.

Limit alcohol consumption.

Avoid contact with tobacco.

Based on these recommendations, I encourage you to design a meal plan that works for you. Changes in diet are unique for each person. For someone who eats a lot of red meat, the first step is to decide how to replace it. Someone else might have to reduce flour and sweets. (In appendix 1,

"Nutrition," you'll find more information to help you focus on what's useful for you.)

Each of us has to find our own path.

> *Wanderer, there is no road; the way is made by walking.*
> —Antonio Machado, *Proverbs and Songs*, Verse XXIX

Antonio understood the importance of adjusting his diet, but he still had doubts about losing weight—which he told me, "has always been hard for me."

I explained to him that being overweight can be the result of imbalances on other levels. As we saw in chapter 4, "Now What?" all dimensions are related. Some people gain weight when they're depressed, for example, and then when they're overweight (or even out of shape), their mood is affected, creating a vicious cycle of depression and further weight gain. If our body being overweight is trying to tell us we're not living in balance, how can we get the message and respond?

Practice for Healthy Living

Do you need support for your diet change?

A **good shopping list** (see Shopping List in appendix 1, "Nutrition") will help you have everything on hand when you start cooking.

Glass containers will allow you to cook large quantities of vegetables and then freeze portions for future meals.

A **cooking class** taught by a health-conscious chef can give you creative ideas.

Living a healthy life is reflected in the body. When we feel we're at the right weight, our self-esteem grows and we feel inclined toward healthier living, caring about what benefits us, and to take better care of ourselves.

Nutrition is related not only to *what we eat* **but also to** *the way we eat.* If we eat healthy foods while in the midst of an emotional crisis, or if we ingest a "healthy" diet in a rigid, demanding way, stress—which creates the opposite result, is generated. When feeling stressed, the body kicks into emergency mode and begins storing as much fat as possible. When we eat while feeling anxious, angry, or in a heated discussion, our digestion and the processing of nutrients are challenged. **It's much healthier to eat in a relaxed and pleasant atmosphere,** taking the time to breathe and calm ourselves before we begin. Religions encourage us to take a moment of silence or prayer before meals. When we're relaxed and at peace, the body metabolizes what we eat in a normal, healthy way.

Antonio was still doubtful. "It stresses me to think so much about food. Do I need to bring lunch with me everywhere I go? Can't I eat with friends when they go out for pizza or fast food?"

We talked about diets. If we're too strict, getting ingredients, preparing meals, deciding whom to eat with, or dealing with the logistics of eating out can be stressful. In Argentina, where I live, eating out is difficult because the traditional cuisine is heavily based on flour (pies, empanadas, pizzas) and meat (we're famous for barbecue). It's the same in the US with so much bread, red meat, and potatoes. We could refuse to eat out so we're not tempted to eat foods that harm us, but spending time with friends is also important. Avoiding enjoyable experiences in order to give sole priority to diet isn't healthy either. It makes no sense to get stressed trying to follow a healthy diet.

I suggested that Antonio try to eat a healthy diet while, at the same time, finding **a balance between nutritious eating and connection with friends.** Gradual changes in diet could help him get used to new flavors (fewer sweets, unfamiliar spices) and could help his intestinal flora and gastrointestinal rhythm get adjusted, to avoid diarrhea or constipation.

It's important to **emphasize the quality** of food. If we limit ourselves to high-quality foods, little by little we'll lose interest in meals and beverages that used to satisfy us. We'll no longer crave ice cream unless it's of a high quality and a flavor we really like. We'll no longer eat a croissant unless it's from a great bakery, and we'll savor it when we do.

Food Is Your Fuel

What kind of fuel are you going to choose today: regular or premium?

In addition to high-quality ingredients, **the way we cook and the environment where the food is prepared are important.** Heat alters food's properties and destroys some vitamins and proteins, so it's sometimes recommended that we eat one-third of our foods raw. When we cook, it's better to boil, bake, steam, or cook on a griddle, and to avoid frying. Some studies have shown that microwaves alter the chemical structure of foods, reducing their nutritive properties.

A meal prepared under stress or in a chaotic atmosphere is not the same as a meal prepared with love. Our grandmother's soup or stew, for example, was much tastier than canned soup! Many people make the effort to keep a pleasant atmosphere in their kitchens by listening to inspiring music or chanting mantras[56] while cooking.

Practice for Healthy Living

Connect with the pleasure of eating, of feeling your body healthy.

The way we store food also affects its quality. Plastic containers transmit unhealthy molecules, such as bisphenol A (BPA), an endocrine disruptor—which means that even at low concentrations, it may cause hormonal system imbalances. BPA is used to produce plastics found in many kitchen containers, bottles, lids, and plastic utensils. Special attention is recommended to prevent babies and toddlers from coming into contact with BPA. Several countries outlaw the use of plastic bottles that have BPA, and it's required in some places, including California, that toy and other manufacturers inform buyers if their products contain BPA.

Practice for Healthy Living

- Choose beverages packaged in non-plastic bottles.
- Look on the bottom of plastic bottles for the recycling code. Avoid bottles identified with numbers 3, 6, and 7.
- If you use plastic containers, don't expose them to the sun or extreme heat because that releases BPA.
- When cooking, use metal or wooden utensils rather than plastic ones.
- Avoid warming food in plastic containers. Use ceramic or glass containers.
- If you use plastic wrap, avoid direct contact with food. You can wrap the food first (or instead) with butcher paper, freezer paper, sandwich paper, or wax paper.
- If you use freezer dividers, make sure they are BPA-free.

We need both discipline and flexibility to change unhealthy habits. It's important to make changes gradually, so we're able to adopt them for life. If we make changes with love, it's easier. We might even influence others.

Eating Turns Food into Life

Sleep

We spend a third of our time sleeping. **A good night's sleep is essential for our health.** Just as we need to satisfy our desire for food, water, and oxygen, we must satisfy our need for sleep.

Several theories try to explain the importance of sleep.[57] One posits that sleep replenishes in the body what is expended while we're awake. Research shows that animals entirely deprived of sleep lose all immune functions and die in a matter of weeks.[58] Sleep gives us the opportunity to **restore and rejuvenate ourselves.** During sleep, we reproduce skin and hair and repair our muscles and all internal systems. Major restorative functions in the body like muscle growth, tissue repair, protein synthesis, and growth hormone release occur mostly during sleep.

Another study found that **sleep correlates to changes in the structure and organization of the brain.** It's known that sleep is essential for brain development during the first years of life, which is the reason infants need to sleep thirteen to fourteen hours per day. Now we see that this is important in adults as well, that sleep deprivation affects our ability to learn and perform certain tasks. It's also believed that during sleep *our brain cleans itself.* While we're awake, the brain produces adenosine, and as it accumulates it makes us feel tired. During sleep, adenosine is eliminated, and we wake up feeling alert. Drinking caffeinated beverages blocks the activity of adenosine in the brain, keeping us alert.

Recent studies show that we **also process emotional experiences during sleep.** Although this research is not yet definitive, we know we're sometimes irritable, hyperreactive, sensitive, and anxious after a bad night's sleep. Chronic sleep deprivation can interfere with the cortex's regulation of the limbic, emotional brain.[59]

Other researchers talk about **connecting with our wise, intuitive, spiritual depths** in the form of a dream or an insight during sleep, having access to information or perspectives not usually accessible to us. When we have a problem, common sense recommends that we "sleep on it."

Although none of the theories about the meaning of sleep is conclusive, scientists do know its benefits. Sleep plays a key role in health because it's involved in the metabolic functioning of the immune system, cognitive functioning (thinking, reasoning, learning, and memory), and other vital processes.

The Doubling Theory of Time

The doubling theory of time described by Jean-Pierre Garnier Malet, a contemporary French physicist, offers a new way to understand the space-time continuum, making "possible the explanation of the mechanics of life, our thoughts and the best possible use of intuitions, instincts and foresight that this doubling makes available to us at every instant."[60]

Based on this theory, falling asleep consciously allows us to reinforce our intuition and change our perception of who we really are.

Practice for Healthy Living

Try this simple exercise before going to sleep.

Once you're in bed with your eyes closed and feeling relaxed, think of some issue you'd like clarified and frame it as an open question, such as, What is my next step toward better health? What is it I'm not seeing that could help my healing? What should I let go of in order to move forward on the path to recovery?

When formulating the question, be confident that the wisest part of you already knows the answer.

The response may come to you in a dream that night or through something you read, hear, see, or even think or imagine in the following days.

Sleep deprivation (not sleeping or not getting enough sleep) is a chronic problem in the modern world. A lack of sleep affects our immune system, putting us on high alert and making us more susceptible to diseases, including cancer. A bad night's sleep affects our mood and cognitive functioning and can increase the risk of an accident. *Chronic* sleep deprivation can affect immunity and metabolism. When we're on alert, cortisol production increases and melatonin decreases. Cortisol is a stress hormone, and its increase makes us more vulnerable to disease, as we saw in chapter 2, "So ... What Is Cancer?" Melatonin is produced by the pineal gland in the brain's depth and regulates sleep and wakefulness. When it's dark, the pineal gland releases more melatonin; it releases less when it's light. Exposure to strong light after the sun goes down or to dim light during the day can affect our melatonin-release cycles. Melatonin has strong antioxidant effects that reverse free radicals' effect, strengthening the immune system, and could have apoptotic (cell death) and anti-angiogenic activity, inhibiting the growth of new blood vessels. Experiments with animals have shown that when they were deprived of sleep, they developed tumors more rapidly.

Going against the biological clock, i.e., being awake at night and asleep during the day, interferes with hormonal cycles. When it's dark out, the body produces melatonin, helping regulate other hormones and maintaining the body's circadian rhythm. Our internal clock plays a key role in the sleep–wakefulness cycle. During sleep, the hormones that help control appetite, metabolism, and the continuous production of glucose to nourish the organs are released. Sleep interruption alters hormone production, appetite,[61] and metabolism and can result in binge eating, especially sweets, even if we've already had enough calories during the day. Bad sleep increases levels of cortisol and insulin, leading to increased blood pressure and glycemia, favoring a pro-inflammatory condition. In addition, since altering the sleep-wakefulness cycle leaves us tired, we might exercise less. The chronic combination of these factors can increase the risk of obesity, diabetes, and cardiovascular disease and eventually bring about an early death.

We don't need as many hours of sleep as we think. In fact, sleeping more than nine hours is also associated with diabetes and cardiovascular disease.[62] **Sleeping six to eight hours a night seems to be the best for most adults, and the time to do so is between 10p.m and 6a.m.**

When we wake up at 3a.m., what should we do? Several practices are recommended, even if you have insomnia due to jet lag or shift work. These are known as *sleep hygiene.*[63]

It can be jarring to be awakened by a loud alarm clock. Try to find a clock that simulates a sunrise, with a light that gradually increases to wake you up naturally.

Getting a good night's sleep requires some preparation during the day.

The bed must be used only to sleep and have sex. If you watch TV, work, or eat in bed, it can make it more difficult to relax and fall asleep.

Exposure to sunlight during the day and darkness at night can increase melatonin production to favor a healthy sleep–wakefulness cycle.

How to Prepare Your Sleep Environment

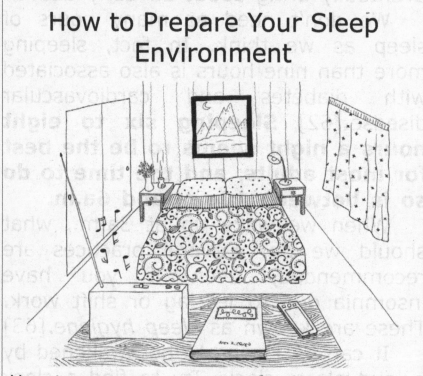

How to prepare your room for a good night's sleep.

It's possible to create a sleep sanctuary, to turn your bedroom into the perfect environment for sleep.

Your bedroom needs to be cool, dark, and quiet. Even the softest light can alter your inner clock and the production of melatonin and serotonin in the pineal gland.

Reduce electromagnetic fields (EMF) in the room; they can alter melatonin levels. It's best to avoid having a television or a computer in your bedroom. If they're there, turn them off an hour before sleeping. If there are other electric devices that could generate electromagnetic fields, such as an alarm clock or a cell phone, especially if it's being charged, keep it at least a yard away from your bed.

Listen to relaxing music, white noise, or the sounds of nature, such as the sea. This can be relaxing and favor sleep. White noise is a random combination of the frequencies the human ear can perceive (between 20 and 20.000 Hz), similar in sound to a hair dryer or a fan. Although there's no scientific explanation why white noise is relaxing, it's frequently used to calm babies and help them sleep.

The simplest explanation is that it masks all other sounds, so a crying baby will stop listening to himself and will allow himself to be calmed down. Aromatherapy and essential oils can also create a relaxing environment.

Exercising at least thirty minutes during the day helps us sleep better. It's best to exercise **early in the morning and outdoors.** Doing so stimulates cortisol secretion, which activates our *alert* mode. If we exercise close to bedtime, it might make it harder to fall asleep.

What we **ingest,** especially in the hours before bedtime, can also affect whether we'll be able to fall asleep easily and sleep well.

- Avoid **caffeinated products** (coffee; black, green, and mate teas; chocolate; soda; and some medicines for cold and flu).
- Avoid **cigarettes** or tobacco products.
- Do not drink **fluids** for two hours before bedtime so you won't have to get up to go to the bathroom.

- Avoid **alcohol.** Although alcohol makes us sleepy, the effect is brief. We'll wake up later, and it will be difficult to get back to sleep.
- For supper, include eggs, nuts, fruits and vegetables, fish or meat. These **proteins** contain an amino acid called tryptophan, which helps us fall asleep.[64]
- Avoid sweets. Sugar in the blood delays sleep. And later, when sugar levels decrease, it can wake us up and make it difficult to fall back asleep.

We sleep about eight hours a day. How can we make these eight hours most effective?

Go to bed early. The body restores most of its energy between 11p.m. and 1a.m.[65] Going to sleep and waking up at the **same time every day** helps the body establish a rhythm that enhances the sleep-wake cycle. **If you take a nap, it's best to do so early;** otherwise, avoid it. Napping late in the day can make it difficult to fall asleep at night.

Establishing a Healthy Sleep–wake Supports a Healthy Life Rhythm

It can be helpful to establish pre-sleep routines to prepare for bed, an hour-long transition period of relaxing activities.

If you can't fall asleep within twenty minutes or if you wake during the night, rather than staying in bed looking at the clock or tossing and turning anxiously, get out of bed and do something relaxing, like light reading or listening to music, keeping lights down, and when you're really tired, go back to bed. In other words, **go to sleep when you're really tired.**

If all else fails, external help may be considered—first, a melatonin supplement and as a final, *temporary* means, a sleeping pill.

Melatonin supplements are less effective than the melatonin we produce naturally. However, research suggests melatonin supplements can help us get to sleep more quickly, especially when we have an altered circadian rhythm, such as when we work at night or suffer from jet lag.

Sleeping pills can cause addiction, and people who take them gradually need higher doses.[66] Research studies indicate that most prescription sleeping pills not only cause fragmented sleep, they also cause amnesia, and when you wake up, you don't remember how bad your sleep really was.[67] They've also been associated with a variety of health risks, including an increased risk of cancer and even death.

Practice for Healthy Living

• Take a warm bath.
• Use the toilet just before getting into bed, to make it less likely you'll wake up during the night to go to the bathroom.
• Wear socks or put a hot water bottle near your feet. Feet often get cold when the body relaxes.
• Read an inspiring or spiritual text to de-stress your mind and to bring you closer to the essence of life.
• Keep a journal. If you tend to have a restless mind around bedtime,

it can be helpful to write down your thoughts, and then put them aside.

• Replace stressful activities (late-night work, watching TV, or discussing emotional issues), which set you in alert mode, with meditation, conscious breathing, or your partner's massage.

• If necessary, wear an eye mask to block light.

Conscious and periodic exercise, good nutrition and hydration, and a thoughtful sleep rhythm give the body vital energy. The way we exchange energy with the environment, through breathing, laughing, and relationships, also affects our energy level (see chapter 9, "Tuning Up").

Our Environment

To be attuned to our environment, we need to activate our senses, keep our bodies clean, and cultivate contact with everything around us. Our senses are the doors or antennae that allow direct contact with the environment.

How to Create Favorable Conditions in Our Environment

Decorate the rooms where you spend most of your day with flowers, art, and pleasing colors to enhance your visual experience.

In rooms where you want to relax, avoid putting anything related to work, responsibilities, or pending tasks that might cause stress or induce guilt.

Play background music and have pleasing fragrances at hand to enhance your experience.

Our environment affects us. Creating order and discarding what we no longer need—e.g., working on a clear desktop and sleeping in an uncluttered bedroom—maximize energy. If our environment is noisy, dirty, or ugly, we're more likely to be on high alert. When our environment is pleasant, it can be easier to relax. Decorators and *feng shui* experts know this and take it into account.

Treat your body as well as you take care of your home or your car. Keep it tidy and clean with conscious breathing and a healthy gastrointestinal rhythm to avoid constipation.

The Importance of Touch

- Allow yourself warm skin contact.
- Choose pleasant-feeling clothes.
- Take bubble baths.
-

Use (paraben-free) body lotion after a shower.[68]

Touch provides the body with important information. Newborns, even when they're well nourished, die if they don't have affectionate contact. Warm skin contact increases relaxation.

Care and stimulation of the body not only makes us feel better, it boosts our immune system. As we've seen, a seed needs favorable conditions to germinate. It's the same with habits and how we care for our body. A revitalized body with a healthy immune system can serve us better than any medical treatment. The next chapter will describe medical treatments that are geared toward eliminating tumors as well as treatments that boost our immune system.

Take-Home Message

The most effective medicine is self-care, awakening our own healing potential.

To change habits, we need to involve our body and provide favorable conditions.

Just as we spend time eating and sleeping, we need to exercise every day.

No amount of exercise can balance a poor diet.

Eating is the way we turn food into life.

Revitalizing the body—a healthy diet, exercise, good sleep, and stress management—is an essential part of any treatment.

Chapter 6

FROM TREATING CANCER TO TREATING THE WHOLE PERSON

Before you know what kindness
really is
you must lose things,
feel the future dissolve in a
moment
like salt in a weakened broth.
What you held in your hand,
what you counted and carefully
saved,
all this must go so you know
how desolate the landscape can be
between the regions of kindness....
Then it is only kindness that makes
sense anymore,
only kindness that ties your shoes
and sends you out into the day to
mail letters and
purchase bread,

> *only kindness that raises its head*
>   *from the crowd of the world to say*
>   *it is I you have been looking for....*

> —NAOMI SHIHAB NYE[1]

Patricia, a successful attorney, came to my office with a friend. She was accustomed to supporting others with their conflicts, but this time it was she who needed care. "Doctor," she said. "I've come to see you because I hear you don't usually recommend surgery. I have lung cancer, and I'm determined not to have surgery. I hope you agree." I looked at Patricia, recognizing that helping her would be a challenge.

Patricia was lucky; her cancer had been detected at an early stage. Most lung cancers are detected late, when a cure option isn't even considered. Conventional medicine had a host of options for someone in her situation.

Fifty percent of those who receive a cancer diagnosis—and up to 90 percent with some kinds of cancer—are cured with conventional medicine. Many kinds of cancer, when diagnosed at an early stage, are curable with surgery.

In specific cases, the positive outcomes of chemotherapy far exceed its temporary, adverse effects. Many patients who have certain leukemias, lymphomas, and testicular cancer, for example, are cured with chemotherapy. The likelihood of a cure is considerably higher when cancer is diagnosed at an early stage. Once it has spread, the chances of a cure decrease significantly. Why wouldn't she consider surgery as the best possibility?

Many people are overloaded with information that makes it difficult to sort it all out and make a coherent decision. There are so many false promises in books and on the internet, radio, and TV that people get confused. **It's important to choose trustworthy, accurate, and appropriate therapists and sources of information.**

I found Patricia's case a challenge because her decision would be so consequential. It could determine whether she would live or succumb to a cancer that had been detected while still operable. I knew I had only one chance—this appointment—to explain the benefits of surgery and help her appreciate how lucky she was that she'd been diagnosed early. If I couldn't persuade her, it was possible she would leave my office and never return.

I told her it wasn't a question of being for or against surgery; I recommend surgery when I consider it necessary. I practice **integrative oncology,** which means I recommend the most advanced therapies found in modern Western medicine while, at the same time, encouraging people to take advantage of psychotherapy and the many *complementary* therapies, including, yoga, meditation, massage, and acupuncture, that focus on **taking care of the whole person, strengthening immunity, and restoring a healthy balance.**[2]

I explained that in her case a cure was possible through surgery, and her cancer could be eliminated and not recur again. Recommending anything other than surgery to Patricia would not have been ethical.

Eastern medicine, e.g., Chinese and Ayurvedic medicine, are excellent for preserving health, but they are not always fast enough when cancer is already established in the body. When a situation is urgent, Western medicine's surgery, radiation, and chemo take effect immediately. When dealing with a starving child, we wouldn't simply try to reverse the causes of malnutrition. If we did so, we'd be putting his life at risk. We'd do all we could to keep him alive first, employing immediate measures to restart nutrition.

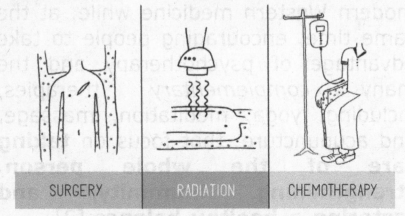

| SURGERY | RADIATION | CHEMOTHERAPY |

Conventional cancer treatments.

I described to Patricia the variety of treatments offered by conventional medicine.

1.　Surgery (localized treatment): the tumor is removed from the body in whole or in part. This may be complemented with radiation and/or chemotherapy.

2. Radiation therapy (localized treatment): uses high-energy rays, such as X-rays, gamma rays, or charged particles. This can be external or internal (implantation in the tumor). Purpose: to remove or shrink cancer cells. The therapy itself is painless, but it may have side effects.

3. Chemotherapy, targeted therapies, hormone therapy, and immunotherapy (systemic treatments): these normally include intravenous (into the vein) or oral administration of medications that travel through the bloodstream. Purpose: to eliminate cancer cells that have spread from the tumor or have installed at a distance (metastasis).

Conventional medicine prescribes one or a combination of these treatments. The treatment and its duration depend on the type and stage of the cancer and the person's general condition. I assured Patricia she would only need surgery from conventional medicine's toolkit. After that, we would investigate what had led her to become ill.

Roberto, the owner of a small shop in the interior of Argentina, arrived at my office with advanced kidney cancer that had metastasized to his bones. He'd been told that, in general, when cancer spreads from its place of origin, it can't be cured, but if he would undergo chemotherapy, bone fortification, and perhaps radiation, it could slow its spread and relieve some of the pain. Roberto had his doubts, "Doctor, is chemotherapy necessary?"

I explained that conventional treatment would be appropriate for his recovery. Because his cancer had spread, he needed a systemic treatment, one that could be distributed throughout his body.

Depending on the kind of cancer, systemic treatments can be based on chemotherapy, targeted therapies, hormone therapy, immunotherapy, or a combination of these. Sometimes we call this treatment *chemo,* but it would be more accurate to refer to it as *systemic treatment.* The type and duration of treatment depend on the goal. Is it intended to cure or to support the recovery process?

When cancer is detected during its early stages, conventional medicine considers that there is a cure option, and the treatment is usually more aggressive and limited in time. In these cases, it's considered more acceptable to tolerate serious adverse effects, since a cure is the intended outcome.

When cancer is more advanced or has spread to other organs, conventional medicine generally doesn't have the tools to cure it. It is treated as a chronic disease, similar to heart disease, diabetes, or hypertension (unusually high blood pressure). A long-term treatment can help control the cancer, reduce pain, relieve symptoms, avoid complications, and sometimes extend a person's life. Because this treatment is not aiming at a cure, aggressive chemotherapies impairing the quality of life are not justified. It makes little sense that as a result of the treatment, a person spends most of his time bedridden, suffering without enjoying life.

We must individualize each treatment, focusing on the person and not on the treatment. Each person is different. It will depend on how they respond to treatment and how the adverse effects impact them.

We can't say that everyone suffering from cancer needs to receive chemotherapy until the last day of their life. Someone in poor health might not be strong enough to undergo a systemic treatment. Or perhaps this person needs a break. Or in light of the person's age and other medical conditions, he or she might decide not to receive the treatment. These decisions are always made by the person with the physician and loved ones, after clearly understanding the possible results of a treatment. Whatever decision is made, the health staff will continue to help the patient stay comfortable, maintaining a life of quality and strengthening the person's immune system to the extent possible.

Sometimes a treatment is a bridge to keep open the possibility of a more promising treatment later on. There are cases of people who had diseases considered incurable at the time, such as chronic myeloid leukemia, melanoma, and kidney cancer, who now, with new chemotherapy drugs known as *targeted therapy,* have years of life ahead instead of weeks. I've seen individuals go from having no hope to trying a new medication, who are still alive many years later.

Roberto started with chemotherapy and a bone fortifier, but he knew the options and prognoses given by conventional medicine were limited. He was not able to travel for our next session, so we met via Skype. "Doctor, what else can I do?" he asked.

I shared my sense that any cancer treatment should include conventional medicine but not be limited to it. Many factors contribute to *cancering,* including food, lifestyle, and psychosocial conditions. Cancer is a process, not an object. We're like a garden or an orchard, not an engine.[3] We can remove tumors through surgery or radiation as though they were weeds, and use chemo or hormone therapy to prevent new tumors, but if we don't irrigate the soil and replenish the ground, the cancerous weeds might return.

From the point of view of integrative medicine, we work the ground using psychotherapy and *complementary* therapies, including diet, exercise, massage, yoga, acupuncture, and meditation, many of which find their origins in Chinese, Ayurvedic, or other traditional medicines.

New research has verified that psychotherapy and *complementary* modalities reduce stress, strengthen immunity, offset factors that give rise to disease, provide emotional clarity, and promote healthy attitudes. Stress-reduction techniques help bring about the relaxation response by stimulating the autonomic parasympathetic nervous system and counteracting the effects of the sympathetic system. As a result, these techniques reduce symptoms and ameliorate some of the adverse effects of treatment, helping provide a better quality of life.

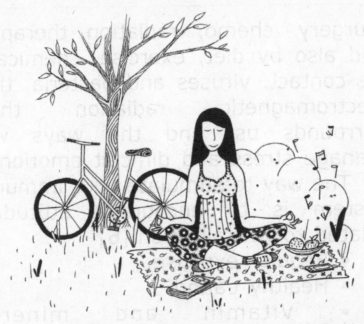

Therapies that help us recover our health.

More and more scientific evidence shows that by stimulating the immune system,[4] *complementary* therapies help mitigate cancer and induce apoptosis, programmed cell death.[5] These therapies are thus used independent of the stage and kind of disease.

Practice for Healthy Living

What can I take to stimulate the immune system?

Our immune system is affected both by cancer and its treatment (surgery, chemo, radiation therapy) and also by diet, exercise, chemicals we contact, viruses and bacteria, the electromagnetic radiation that surrounds us, and the ways we manage stress and difficult emotions.

The way to stimulate your immune system is to encourage attitudes related to revitalization.[6]

- Regular exercise.
- Healthy eating.
- Vitamin and mineral supplements, as necessary.
- Sound sleep.
- Stress management techniques, like conscious breathing, meditation, yoga, and Reiki. There is evidence that meditation techniques improve immunological parameters.
- Support groups.[7] Not all groups use the same techniques, and some are more beneficial than others. The most beneficial groups are those that strengthen immunity and reduce stress.
- Avoid tobacco.
- Avoid exposure to midday sun.

- Laughing, dancing, and singing stimulate the immune system. There are techniques such as laughter therapies or yoga of laughter designed to stimulate laughter. YouTube videos show these techniques in practice and will make you laugh.
- Avoid pollution. Environmental pollutants such as plastics, latex, fertilizers and herbicides like glyphosate,[8] preservatives, flavoring and other chemicals in food, etc., tax the immune system.

Therapies like acupuncture and reflexology stimulate the immune system and produce a state of relaxation. Quality-assured, natural supplements, such as aromatherapy products, homeopathic products, and phytopharmaceuticals, help strengthen our immune system. An integrative physician can suggest which product might be best for you and give advice if some might interact in a negative way with other treatments.

Some personality characteristics (low self-esteem, self-critical capacity, and negative thoughts) and forms of conduct (toxic relationships and negative reactions) suppress the immune system and bring it into a *cancering* mode. Psychotherapy is advisable, preferably a therapy that involves the body, provided that it's part of an overall integrative approach.

Other support measures that stimulate the immune system can be provided by medical systems with holistic approaches, for example anthroposophic medicine, homeopathy, Ayurvedic medicine, and Chinese medicine.

Considering the benefits shown by *complementary* therapies, **integrative support, including these kinds of therapies, is absolutely necessary in all cases.**

Only *complementary* therapies that have been proven safe and effective are recommended. It is important that **therapies be managed by trained therapists with expertise in cancer patients.** There are precautions to be taken in relation to the disease and to the treatment being provided. For example, when massaging, excessive pressure should not be exerted on those with bone metastasis or a tendency to excessive bleeding, e.g., someone who has few platelets as a result of chemotherapy.

Those coming for medical advice along with their families need the care of doctors, nurses, psychologists, and other therapists with an integrative approach. All these practitioners need to know the benefits of conventional treatment and of *complementary* therapies and should be able to guide people to receive the best personalized treatment.[9] Ideally, they should all work at the same institution to provide good communication and support to the patients and their families.

Alternative? Complementary? Conventional?

What are the differences between *conventional*, *alternative*, and *complementary* medicine? The primary distinction is whether an alternative modality is used *instead* of or as a *complement* to what we regard as conventional medicine.

The greatest risk of **alternative therapies** is if they are practiced *in lieu of* surgery and/or chemotherapy in situations when rejecting one of these conventional modalities might mean losing the opportunity to be cured.

Many people who could be cured by a conventional treatment reject it and instead resort exclusively to alternative therapies. When they discover that the alternative therapy did not cure them, it can be too late. This might have been the case with Steve Jobs. He suffered from pancreatic neuroendocrine cancer, which when detected in its early stages, is generally curable with surgery. According to media reports, he undertook alternative therapy treatments, and lost a significant amount of weight. The tumor grew, but when he was open to removing it surgically, it was too late for him to be cured.

Complementary medicine means treatments that *accompany* conventional treatments. They are called *complementary* because they are considered adjuncts to what we call *conventional medicine* in the West. In the East, these kinds of therapies, e.g., massage, meditation, and acupuncture, are part of traditional Ayurvedic and Chinese medicine.

There are many cases showing that *complementary* treatments are as relevant as conventional treatment. Take, for example, the practice of regular exercise in certain persons suffering from colon cancer, who had been appropriately treated with surgery and chemotherapy. The exercise reduces even further the likelihood of cancer recurring, thus increasing life expectancy.[10]

In my opinion, it is not advisable to use the terms *conventional* treatment (chemotherapy, surgery, radiation) and *non-conventional* or *complementary* treatment, since these terms imply that the *complementary* treatment is less important than the conventional one. For all these reasons, I will refer to all conventional therapies that aim to remove cancer directly as **anticancer treatments.** And I will refer to all *complementary* therapies that "strengthen the ground"—allowing the body itself to search for the way to mitigate cancer—as therapies *aimed to strengthen the immune system and the PNIE network.* In fact, most modern immuno-therapies are based on the strategy of strengthening and activating the immune system's cells to attack the tumors.[11]

"I met a healer who says he only needs to strengthen the ground," Roberto insisted, *"and that I can cure my cancer only with energy healing. He told me not to undergo chemotherapy because it would debilitate me."*

I told him that I know there are many healers who are against chemotherapy. They recommend that people not undergo any chemo treatments whatsoever and to cure themselves with only energy healing, homeopathy, Chinese medicine, etc. Extreme positions are not the solution. As Buddhist wisdom states, the key is in the middle way.[12]

Just as surgery is not appropriate for every medical condition—e.g., a bad cold—we can't expect to cure cancer only with homeopathy, energy healing, or healthy food. **Anticancer treatments** address what needs immediate attention, but in general they alone will not impact the root cause. **Therapies intending to strengthen the immune system,** though they take more time, help reverse the imbalances suffered by our energetic body (see chapter 9, "Tuning Up"). Treating the causes frequently stops cancers from recurring and prevents the development of new ones.

Anticancer treatment may not only buy time until there is a new and more effective medication, but it can be a bridge to a new way of life. Like a crutch, chemo might control the disease and allow the person to continue living a normal life.

Some people with cancer discover in the healing process a path of personal growth and spiritual openness, leading them to make outstanding progress in fighting the disease, exceeding the statistics.[13] The most extreme cases have achieved spontaneous healing or regression, the disappearance of tumors even without anticancer medical treatment. There is reliable documentation of **spontaneous healings.** Though rare, they do actually take place.[14]

"Then the healer was right! Many people are cured with energy healing, aren't they?" Roberto insisted.

I explained to him that frequently, people whose cancer goes into remission attribute it to therapies like Reiki or a special diet. I encouraged him to be skeptical about any therapy that *promises* healing, e.g. "I was cured by such-and-such." Not everyone who tries that modality overcomes their illness. Generally, spontaneous healings like these are few and far between. Although the body's innate intelligence knows how to contain and even reverse disease, only rarely can someone activate self-healing capabilities and overcome a life-threatening illness through that alone.

In my opinion, a spontaneous regression has to do with **restoring a new order** in the complex system that we are and in which we're immersed. It's important to focus on the person as a whole, *in a holistic way,* to address physical, mental, emotional, spiritual, and social needs. Therapies that strengthen the immune system do it by restoring a healthy balance. It's this *recovery of balance* that allows the immune system and the PNIE network to work properly, helping the cancer disappear and restoring the person's vitality.

These holistic approaches recognize that the human being is a complex system and that changes in one element affect the whole person. In a garden, to produce an azalea blossom we need moisture, partial shade, and acidic pH soil to achieve the dynamic balance that promotes blooming. In the same way, we must **provide the appropriate conditions** to help someone regain balance. We must help that person improve nutrition, remove toxins, release accumulated stress, modify negative thought patterns, express and release emotions, reorganize strained relationships within the family or social network, and align with a meaningful life.

Healing depends on being able to reverse the conditions that led to disease and allow the multidimensional being that we are to leap forward in health. This leap implies a broadening of consciousness, not just following one therapy or another blindly. **The one who cures is the person, not the therapy.**[15]

In a complex system, small changes can produce large results. For this reason, it's difficult to predict someone's progress. Each person's path is personal and unique. No one can know for certain how long it will take someone to heal or how long he or she is going to live.

Elisa, a woman devoted to family and home, came to me with a localized breast cancer. She'd been advised to undergo surgery followed by radiation and adjuvant chemotherapy, which means applying chemo after all the known and visible cancer was removed surgically and with radiation therapy. She found it challenging to follow the daily radiation dosage, and when she began chemo, she suffered from anticipatory nausea and worried she was no longer strong enough to face the treatment.

Elisa seemed to be on permanent alert, and I wondered if this was because of the cancer or if there were additional stress factors. Following the multidimensional approach, I learned that her husband had resumed drinking in excess, leading to violent behavior. In the past when he was drunk, he would beat her.

Obviously, this amplified the symptoms. For example, she experienced nausea even before receiving chemotherapy. She wasn't sleeping well, which further suppressed her immune system and PNIE network. All of this affected her health and kept her from following the recommended treatment.

It's important to take into account the anticancer treatment *itself* as well as its effects on the immune system's recovery and to remove all the *cancering* factors in order to reestablish healthy conditions. Although it can be difficult to start an anticancer treatment while undergoing psychotherapy, changing diet, increasing exercise, and learning stress management, with a good guide it is possible.

It's also important that the oncologist, together with the health team, evaluate all these dimensions to see which factors are playing the leading role in the persistence of the *cancering* mode. If the dominant factors are unhealthy habits, like overeating, sedentariness, or poor sleep, improving these dimensions can be a good start. If the most evident factor is work-related stress based on real issues or a failure to face work maturely, this would be the first factor to address. If the main problem is a toxic relationship, this is the most important factor to deal with at the outset. In Elisa's case, an integrative approach would value her medical treatment *equally* with finding solutions to her unhealthy relationship. Each person is different, and the recommendations depend on the situation.

María, a forty-two-year-old graphic designer, came to me following breast cancer surgery. She'd been advised to have radiation following surgery, and when she found out the treatment meant going to the radiotherapy center daily for five weeks, she worried she couldn't do it and go to work, too.

I agreed with her that organizing her time to have treatment every day would be the most cumbersome part of the radiation therapy. It was important, I suggested, to remember that the treatment would last only five weeks and for her to see the situation in context, that this would be a relative inconvenience compared to a recurrence of cancer.

I suggested she arrive at the radiation appointments ahead of time and to plan on a pleasant activity every day and not just focus on the disease. For example, she could meet a friend and spend time together before or after the treatment or schedule a reflexology session following treatment. María agreed to meet a good friend she couldn't ordinarily meet often, and because of the meaningful conversations they had, the time in the waiting room passed quickly. These strategies helped her tolerate the treatment better.

Now, let's see how to start an integrative treatment, which means anticancer treatment together with therapies to strengthen the immune system.

Diagnostic Procedures

The period of diagnostic procedures is difficult and filled with uncertainty. As soon as you feel there's a possibility of cancer, fear, anxiety and regression are triggered, which result in a tsunami of stress hormones released within the body. Generally, getting test results takes more time than you'd wish. Two or three weeks, or longer, might pass before you receive an accurate diagnosis. During this time, though a cancer diagnosis has not been confirmed, you start to suffer—sleep disruption, anxiety, lack of concentration, fear, and anguish—all symptoms that prevent you from functioning with ease.

It can be helpful to employ stress management techniques during this period—breathing exercises or meditation, for example. When it's possible, going for a walk can help us cope with anxiety, and it stimulates the immune system. A session of reflexology can help, or a salt bath. These practices can help counteract stress, keep an internal balance, and live in this difficult time in the best way possible. Once the diagnosis is confirmed and the treatment plan is in place, many people are better able to face the situation, and their anxiety levels diminish.

The Waiting Room

Sitting in the waiting room can be stressful in itself, whether you're waiting for a diagnostic procedure, a treatment, or a medical exam. You might like to bring some soothing music, a meditation, or guided relaxation to listen to while you're waiting. This helps reduce anxiety and balances the sense of dread. Some people take adult coloring books, e.g., a mandala sketchbook and some color pencils, to express their creativity. If the doctor is running late, you can ask if his office will call when they're ready and go outside for a walk, a sit in the sun, or a nearby coffee shop. Think about what might help you enter the appointment in the best condition, able to tolerate the treatment and leave without feeling unduly depleted.

Preparing for Surgery and Recovery

The effects of surgery and the recovery period afterward depend on the kind of surgery, the area of the body, how deep it is, and how prepared you are beforehand.

For any kind of surgery, always consult with doctors who have expertise in that particular operation. Studies of those who had to undergo complicated surgeries show that the results correlate with the number of operations in the facility and the surgeon's expertise.

Practice conscious breathing.

If you'd like, close your eyes.

Follow the flow of air as it enters your nostrils, goes down your throat and into your lungs, and say to yourself, "In," or "I am breathing in."

While exhaling, follow the flow of air back, and say to yourself, "Out," or "I am breathing out."

Repeat this ten times.

Before opening your eyes, observe how you feel. Has anything changed? How is your body? How are your thoughts?

This exercise has no side effects! You can practice it several times a day.[16]

The condition of the person undergoing surgery is also important. Many surgeons postpone surgery when the patient has extreme fear because they know those surgeries are more likely to get complicated.

Prepare yourself by practicing deep relaxation or self-hypnosis exercises for at least a few days before your operation to arrive more relaxed. The mood in the operating room is also important. Some surgeons, assistants, anesthesiologists, and surgical technologists choose the music to listen to during the surgery, and many of them meditate or pray before each surgery.

For a prompt recovery, it's important to get out of bed and walk according to the surgeon's instructions, and to continue practicing stress management techniques during the days following surgery.

Some people recommend arnica to speed the healing of wounds after surgery. However, be mindful. Arnica interferes with anticoagulant medications that are usually used with patients who must rest after surgery.

The Adverse Effects of Radiation Therapy

Radiation treatment is like having an X-ray or a CT scan. In itself, it's painless. The inconvenience is adjusting to the rhythm of going for treatments every day. Common side effects are irritation of the radiated area and fatigue.

Depending on the area where the radiation is applied, it might affect the skin or mucous membranes.[17] There are natural therapies that can ease these adverse effects and prevent complications.

The skin of the radiated area and the adjacent areas will tend to dehydrate and become more sensitive. It's always recommended to keep that area exposed to fresh air but to avoid direct sun exposure during treatment and for some months after, whenever possible. Even when the affected area is exposed to the sun, it has to be protected with sunscreen and moisturizers. Aloe vera, chamomile, calendula, and rose hips help cleanse, soothe, heal, and regenerate the skin. Aloe vera can be applied on the skin as a gel or resin, rose hips applied as an oil, calendula applied as an oil or added to bathwater, and chamomile as an infusion for bathing. Apply any of these products *after* each radiation session, since the skin must be absolutely clean for the treatment.

Radiation in the head and neck areas may produce inflammation of the mouth and throat, known as mucositis. To prevent mucositis or reduce its severity:

> • Keep your mouth clean and healthy. Brush your teeth with a soft toothbrush using a good brushing technique. Gargle with saltwater.
> • Be sure to have dentures repaired and cavities filled to avoid wounds.
> • Avoid alcohol, smoking, and spicy, very hot, and acidic foods.
> • Suck ice cubes (cryotherapy)[18] while undergoing chemotherapy.

Radiation therapy may disrupt saliva production and cause dry mouth. Acupuncture can help with this.

After surgery and radiation in the armpit due to breast cancer, an edema (swelling) may appear in the arm. Lymphatic drainage helps soothe it.

Radiation treatment can produce extreme exhaustion that is difficult to overcome, even with rest. Maintaining a moderate physical activity level during the weeks of treatment is important to help avoid this. How much physical activity is wise varies from person to person. This must be supervised by professionals and adapted to each person according to the possibilities and their preferences.

Though vitamin E may prevent fibrosis or scarring from radiation therapy, the use of high-dose antioxidants during treatment is controversial. They may interfere with the effects of radiation and of some chemotherapies.[19] The decision whether to take antioxidants and at what dosage must be made with your doctor, taking into account your traits, the intention and kind of treatment, and the risk of side effects.

Practice for Healthy Living

Anticipate that you might be fatigued, that your skin will be chafed, that you won't feel great. Review your schedule of activities for the treatment period, and only keep appointments that are really necessary. Leave time for exercise and long rest periods to conserve your energy and contribute to your health.

It's important to avoid taking substances that haven't been investigated and might interfere with radiation therapy, possibly increasing its toxicity or reducing its effectiveness.

Chemotherapy's Adverse Effects

There are many kinds of chemotherapy, and each has its own characteristic side effects. Classic chemotherapies indiscriminately impact all the cells that are multiplying. As cancer cells multiply rapidly, chemotherapy will kill them. But it also kills other body cells that are actively multiplying, such as hair root cells; mucous membrane cells that coat the inside of the digestive tract from the mouth to the end of the intestines; and bone-marrow cells, where blood is produced.

Classic chemotherapy's short-term adverse effects may include nausea and vomiting, reduced appetite, hair loss, and mouth sores. Not all chemotherapies cause hair loss. Even some of the effects feared in the past, like nausea and vomiting, are now preventable or treatable with new medications. Since chemo affects bone marrow cells, the number of cells in the blood is reduced. Due to the lack of white blood cells, the risk of infection may increase. If there's a reduction in platelets, there might be a greater tendency to bleed or bruise after minor injuries. Anemia may occur, with tiredness, shortness of breath, and pallor due to the reduced number of red blood cells.

Modern chemotherapies, like targeted therapies and immunotherapy, affect cancer cells and the immune system differently from the way they affect the rest of the body. In general, they have fewer adverse effects than classic chemotherapies, but they're sometimes difficult to administer. Although they do not produce as much nausea, vomiting, or hair loss, they may affect the skin or the gastrointestinal tract, produce high blood pressure, and create wound-healing problems.

Some individuals tolerate the same chemotherapy treatment more easily than others, depending on their general condition. Someone who maintains a healthy weight and is in good psychophysical health will probably tolerate chemo better than someone less fit.

Chemotherapy's adverse effects are not only due to the absorption of medication by the body. Receiving chemo affects us mentally and emotionally as well, producing fear and anguish. Many people suffer from anticipatory nausea *before* receiving the medication. If the environment where the treatment is administered is unpleasant, amplified by a room full of others who are also suffering, that can add to chemo's bad rap. Luckily, many compassionate nurses help make the experience less unpleasant.

Is Chemotherapy Worse Than Cancer Itself?

In view of the difficulty of treatment, the uncertainty of the results, and the side effects, people become discouraged and have doubts about chemotherapy, wondering if it's worth it.

Although it's true that chemotherapy causes side effects, generally they disappear after treatment. Lost hair, for example, grows back. And at times symptoms of the disease are thought to be adverse effects of chemo.

Many kinds of cancer can be cured with chemotherapy. Apprehension about side effects can cause us to underestimate chemo's benefits, missing a chance for a cure.

Preparing for chemo sessions is important. Many people tolerate treatment better if, during the session or even in the waiting room, they listen to pleasant music or practice a guided meditation. Connecting with an artistic work, painting or coloring mandalas, reading a book, or listening to music can help you connect more deeply with yourself, as can avoiding conversations that drain your energy. Talking about your suffering, for example, might not be a beneficial use of your time. When you feel vulnerable, select who you want to be with, what you want to talk about, and conserve your energy to advance in the course of treatment and recovery.

There are natural ways to prevent and treat nausea and vomiting. Ginger prevents nausea, and a protein-rich diet with added ginger may reduce post-chemo nausea. Techniques related to mind-body medicine and relaxation techniques, breathing exercises, meditations, guided visualizations, music therapy, acupuncture, and reflexology can also help relieve nausea, vomiting, and tiredness. These techniques also alleviate anxiety, insomnia, and pain and stimulate the immune system. It's a good idea to include one or more of these techniques before, during, or after your chemotherapy sessions.

One of the most dreaded side effects of chemotherapy is hair loss since it has a strong psychological and social impact, particularly among women and children. It becomes a visible reminder of the disease and produces a feeling of vulnerability, shame, and loss of identity. Others notice our hair loss, making some social interactions difficult. Even though times are changing and shaven heads can be fashionable, the social pressure is still potent.

How to Cope with Hair Loss?

Cold caps and scalp cooling systems may help some women keep some or quite a bit of their hair during chemotherapy.[20]

When chemotherapy might produce hair loss, it's sometimes recommended to cut your hair as short as possible, especially if it's been long, so the effect of becoming bald is less pronounced. Knowing what you'd like and making a decision in advance can help you cope.

Many people wear wigs, scarves, or hats during this period, not just for social reasons but to protect themselves and stay warm, especially in cool weather.

There are organizations like Look Good Feel Better[21] that teach women how to use a scarf and how to apply makeup to create a self-image that makes them feel most comfortable.

How Can We Lessen the Side Effects of Hormone Therapy?

Hormone therapy is used to treat some kinds of breast and prostate cancer. It can produce side effects in both women and men, including tiredness, decrease in libido, hot flashes, gastrointestinal disorders, increase or reduction of appetite, and hair thinning.

Regular exercise or taking rests during the day may help reduce tiredness and ensure a good night's sleep.

Reducing or eliminating coffee, dark tea, nicotine, and alcohol can reduce hot flashes or help you cope with them. It can also be helpful to keep your environment cool, drink iced beverages, and use warm rather than hot water for baths and showers.

Hot flashes are the result of lack of estrogen in women and lack of testosterone in men. Replacement of these hormones could relieve the symptoms, but it isn't advisable to replace hormones in those who have suffered breast or prostate cancer, since that could reactivate the cancer cells. It's uncertain whether the estrogens derived from plants, e.g., phytoestrogens, or those found in soy plants, produce the same effect. It's been found that Asian women suffer less from hot flashes than Western women, which has been attributed to a higher consumption of soy products. Studies have been carried out with phytoestrogens, products derived from soybeans, to see if they reduce hot flashes. However, these studies on Western women, who are not accustomed to soy consumption, have been inconclusive. Therefore, the recommendation is not to consume more phytoestrogens than before and even to avoid them.

Some medications or supplements such as vitamin E can be used to relieve hot flashes, but a doctor should be consulted. Guided visualizations and acupuncture also produce favorable results. Each person should explore what helps him or her.

Hormone therapy may lead women to stop menstruating and cause other symptoms of menopause. Besides hot flashes and a decrease in libido, you may experience vaginal dryness. Lubricants can be really useful.

Other side effects might include headaches, mood swings, weight gain, muscle or joint pain. For osteoarticular (bone-and-joint) pain, exercise such as walking, cycling, or lifting moderate weights can be a good resource. Acupuncture helps alleviate the pain brought about by some hormone therapies administered to women, namely aromatase inhibitors.[22]

These are some basic guidelines to help you implement an integrative approach during anticancer treatment. Through investigation, you might find other things that are useful for you. Information on the internet can be comprehensive, although sources vary greatly. Use caution, and consult with your doctor. (In appendix 2, "Frequently Asked Questions About Treatment," you'll find other information I've found reliable.)

Beyond the anticancer treatment and the focus on stimulating the immune system, cancer is an invitation to learn about healthy nutrition and therapies providing well-being and to pursue a medical path perhaps unknown before. It impels people to explore new worlds, know themselves better, become aware of new ways of living and of what is beneficial and what is harmful, and enter a path toward the unknown. Cancer forces people to question their lives and take responsibility for it. Each of us will find our own answer.

Take-Home Message

Integrative oncology includes anticancer treatment and other therapies that focus on taking care of the person, strengthening the immune system, and restoring a healthy balance.

Integrative support can help everyone.

It's important to choose experienced therapists and reliable information.

Personalized treatment focuses on the person and not on the treatment.

The one who brings about a cure is the person, not the therapy.

> **Cancer is an invitation to take responsibility for how we want to live.**

Chapter 7

THE TREASURE HUNT

Listen, what we see before us is just one tiny part of the world. We get in the habit of thinking, this is the world, but that's not true at all. The real world is a much darker and deeper place than this, and much of it is occupied by jellyfishes. We just happen to forget all that. Don't you agree? Two-thirds of the earth's surface is ocean, and all we can see of it with the naked eye is the surface: the skin. We hardly know anything about what's beneath the skin.
—HARUKI MURAKAMI, *THE WIND-UP BIRD CHRONICLE*

Rocío, a thirty-five-year-old designer, came to my office agitated after quarreling with her parents. After having chemo, she'd gone into remission from acute leukemia and she was eager to improve her health and discover new ways of looking at her life. But once again, she'd lost her temper that morning and was feeling guilty and distressed. "Laura, this is who I am. In the same way I'm a blonde, I'm short-tempered. Every time my parents touch where it hurts, I explode!" She was trying to justify herself.

I sat beside her hoping to engage in a deeper conversation. I asked if her body was the same body she'd had when she was seven. She pictured the seven-year-old version of her body, the twenty-year-old version, and her current body. I told her that not one cell of her twenty-year-old body was a part of her now. Every cell had been replaced.[1] This helped Rocío see we are constantly changing, even though we are under the illusion that we're exactly the same person. We were beginning a treasure hunt. Now she understood the importance of not seeing ourselves as static.

The Body Is Like a River

In *Quantum Healing,* Deepak Chopra reminds us that the body is constantly changing: "With each breath that you take, it changes the river of atoms that is your body."

With each inhalation and exhalation, we are exchanging molecules with the environment.

Our body is constantly reshaping. It's formed by trillions of cells. Billions are dying, and within each cell molecules coexisting in a given moment produce thousands of biochemical reactions. There is no constant substance in the body.[2]

Outside and inside our body, everything is also unfolding continuously. Like a flower that closes at sunset and opens at midday, when we see it as only closed or only blooming, we see an illusion. We perceive two different fixed statuses and don't see the imperceptible movement.

Is it True Our Body Renews Every Seven Years?

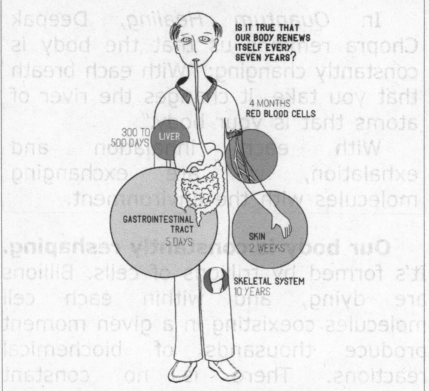

IS IT TRUE THAT OUR BODY RENEWS ITSELF EVERY SEVEN YEARS?

4 MONTHS
RED BLOOD CELLS

300 TO 500 DAYS   LIVER

GASTROINTESTINAL TRACT
5 DAYS

SKIN
2 WEEKS

SKELETAL SYSTEM
10 YEARS

Is it true our body renews every seven years?

Though it is true that most of our body is under constant renewal, according to studies with carbon-14 dating,[3] this assertion is not accurate. Certain cells die; others regenerate. Each cell has its own rhythm: some cells live only days, others months, and yet others years.

Cells inside our digestive system live approximately five days, the superficial layer of the epidermis regenerates every two weeks, red blood cells live approximately four months, liver cells live 300–500 days, the skeleton renews every ten years. Many brain cells renew, though some neurons seem to survive our entire life.

In addition, we're balancing ourselves on a planet that's constantly rotating "around" the sun, participating in a planetary dance. And the whole solar system is traveling through space at high speed. Every moment, though we may have the sense of standing still, we're moving in space at about 43,500 miles/hour, aboard Spaceship Earth.

Did You Know That the Earth Does Not Orbit "Around" the Sun?

We see the solar system as isolated and think planets rotate around the sun in elliptical orbits. But what happens when we observe the solar system within the universe?

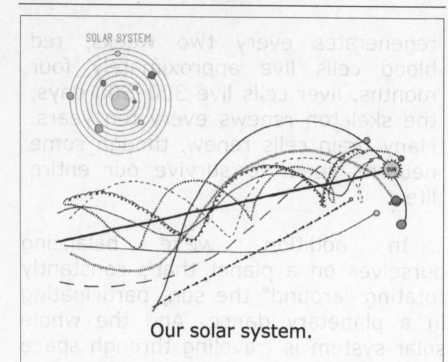

Our solar system.

Recent studies show that while the sun is moving through the universe, it takes along all the planets, which trail behind the sun in a helical path. When we place the solar system in this context, the meaning changes.[4]

If we are continuously moving and changing, how can we stand still? Like a tightrope walker, we need to counterbalance, to flow with movements.

When we face a challenging situation, we need to stay flexible to make the most appropriate decision in each moment, avoiding a mere reaction.

If we simply activate already-known patterns, we remain in a trauma vortex. Unhappy experiences accumulate and become a load and a limitation. Like the iron balls attached to prisoners' ankles, they limit our ability to move with agility, and we're more prone to lose our balance and get sick.

I explained to Rocío that we're anchored to a certain identity, but that's an illusion. We're changing constantly. If we feel tied to an image, we can't move freely, counterbalance, or keep our balance, and we'll fall down. Life is a continuous adaptation to whatever comes our way. **Dancing with the flow of life brings health and joy to body and soul.**

Practice for Healthy Living

Take a few minutes to reflect and write in a journal:

What is holding you back?

What is keeping you from entering the flow of your life?

Life Is Movement

During my consultation with Rocío, we practiced a breathing exercise to help her experience the continuous movement in her own body. When we finished, she told me, "I feel renewed. I can feel the energy coursing through my body."

I was happy to see Rocío connecting with her body, able to feel the effects of conscious breathing. It was a direct experience and therefore "true." She was moving along on the "treasure hunt," finding new clues.

I explained to her that our physical body is "condensed energy" and what she was feeling was *vital energy,* also a part of the body. Most of the time, we don't pay attention to our energetic body. We can't see it, but it's there. Have you ever been in love, felt rage, or tracked a thought? Love, rage, and thinking can't be measured, but they're a part of us just as our liver, our feet, and the color of our eyes are.

Visible Spectrum

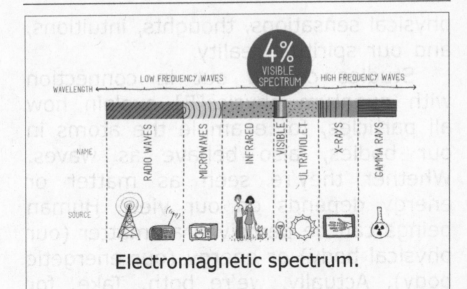

Electromagnetic spectrum.

We are a light spectrum. The physical body is visible to the human eye, but what we can see represents just 4 percent of reality.

Classical physics posits that objects are material bodies with mass and weight, attracted to one another by the force of gravity. This viewpoint appeared in the seventeenth century with Newton, who saw an apple falling from a tree and laid the foundation for the law of universal gravitation.

But from the beginning of the twentieth century, quantum physics has invited us to remove the veil and look beyond. According to quantum physics, vital energy is also a fact, as are physical sensations, thoughts, intuitions, and our spiritual reality.

Studies carried out in connection with quantum physics[5] explain how all particles, for example the atoms in our bodies, also behave as waves. Whether they're seen as matter or energy depends on our view. Human beings can be perceived as matter (our physical body) or energy (our energetic body). Actually, we're both. Take, for example, a lightbulb. When it's turned off, we see only the glass and metal filaments, which are a part of it. When it's on, we see the light that spreads all around. The lightbulb is all of that. Depending on conditions, we'll see different elements.

What we normally call our *body* is our physical body—matter. Cells (matter) are the bricks. Yet the structure of the physical body is formed by thoughts, emotions, sensations, and feelings, which are not made up of matter, but of energy and information. Our beliefs form the foundation. Our memories and thoughts form the scaffolding. Taken as a whole, these are known as the *energetic body*. We generally focus on the physical body, but as the Little Prince says, "The essential is invisible to the eyes."

It was hard for Rocío to face the many challenges facing her, and this was reflected in her relationships. The next time she came into my office, she was upset. She told me she'd had an argument with her partner. I asked her to sit down, close her eyes, breathe deeply, and feel her body. When I asked what was in her mind, she described a frank conversation she imagined having with her partner that night: "The last time we met, you told me the same thing. How can I trust you?"

Body and Soul

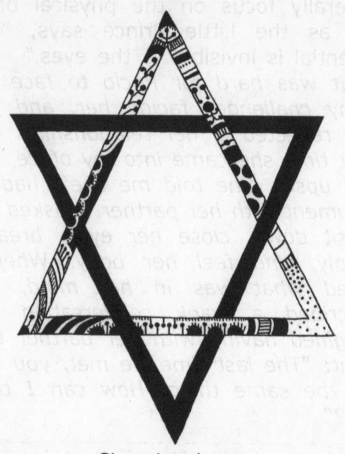

Six-pointed star.

The connection between the physical and energetic bodies, or between the Earth and the sky, has been represented in different ways in different cultures. In the six-pointed star, the lower triangle represents the body, which becomes subtler as it binds to the soul. The upper triangle represents the soul, materializing itself and inhabiting the body.

Once Rocío calmed down, we used the experience to learn how we are in multiple times and places simultaneously. During our conversation, Rocío saw that (1) her body was in my office, (2) her emotions were in the past, in the situation she'd left at home that morning—her stomach was still in a knot, and (3) her mind was soaring into the future, planning a response for the argument she anticipated having that night. Rocío realized how out of alignment she was, that her being had multiple dimensions, each in a different space and time.

Our physical body tends to move more slowly than our energetic body, which is lighter. Thus, at any given moment, they might be out of synch. Practicing conscious breathing, Rocío was able to bring all her parts to the here and now, giving her a feeling of calm and well-being, a sense of gaining control of the situation and trust in her ability to face challenges as they arise.

She had discovered the third clue on her treasure hunt.

Our Energetic Body Travels and Brings Back Information to Our Physical Body

Every particle of the universe has a corpuscular and a wave component, *doubled* into a physical and an energetic body.

One way to see how our energetic body functions draws from the experience of pilots in jet planes. When the plane accelerates sharply, the pilot can *black out,* losing consciousness.[6] This can be described as the energetic body leaving the physical body. Today we can experience something similar in the simulators found in places like Disney World, during which we might experience nausea.

According to Dr. Jean-Pierre Garnier Malet, our information-containing energetic body is our wave component traveling at the speed of light to find information. It then returns to give the information to the physical body. The fact that we're largely made of water allows the information to be transmitted throughout our body instantaneously.[7]

Practice for Healthy Living

Put the book down and take a few minutes.

Your body is in the now.

But where is your mind?

And your emotions?

Write down what you notice.

To connect with the now, the body is our best ally.

And breathing is our best guide.

Most of the time we are living in multiple dimensions, which are not synchronized. This might sound "esoteric," but it is real. Though we usually identify with our mind and thoughts, our life is unfolding on multiple levels simultaneously.

The idea that we have an energetic body was new to Rocío, and she was open and interested in learning about it. "I've never heard about this," she said, and asked me to explain more.

Our energetic body is the invisible packaging that encloses and gives life to our physical body. In some cultures, it's called the *aura,* an energy field with a luminous rainbow that radiates around us like a halo that's invisible to most human beings.

Within the energetic body, we can identify several levels, or bodies, as we saw in chapter 4, "Now What?" Observers throughout human history have described this in various ways. Some base their descriptions on the seven bodies or principles; others describe five. The point is that the energetic or subtle body has multiple levels that continuously give us information about our daily experiences. Picture Russian nesting dolls (*matryoshka*) of decreasing size placed one inside the other to get a sense of these levels functioning together.

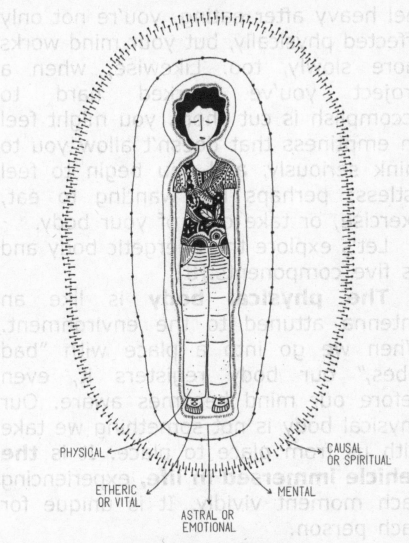

PHYSICAL

CAUSAL OR SPIRITUAL

ETHERIC OR VITAL

MENTAL

ASTRAL OR EMOTIONAL

Our different bodies.

Actually, they're not isolated. It isn't a body inside another body—in a physical way. They're interwoven, interacting, and molding with each other continuously, yet each body maintains its own identity. For example, when you feel heavy after eating, you're not only affected physically, but your mind works more slowly, too. Likewise, when a project you've worked hard to accomplish is cut short, you might feel an emptiness that doesn't allow you to think seriously, and you begin to feel listless; perhaps not wanting to eat, exercise, or take care of your body.

Let's explore the energetic body and its five components.[8]

The physical body is like an antenna attuned to the environment. When we go into a place with "bad vibes," our body registers it, even before our mind becomes aware. Our physical body is not something we take with us from place to place. It is **the vehicle immersed in life,** experiencing each moment vividly. It is unique for each person.

The etheric or vital body is a thin layer that covers the physical body and is connected to it, like a silhouette. The vital body gives the physical body life and fosters its growth. It's the *qi* in Chinese medicine and *prana* in Ayurvedic medicine. The difference between a living body and a dead one is the presence or absence of the vital body. The vital body **contains the molds, or morphic fields, that serve as reference or information for the physical body** from which the structures of the physical body are formed.[9] For example, after a fracture, the vital body provides the mold to rebuild the affected bone. Each vital body is unique and is molded according to experiences lived, which leave imprints.

The astral or emotional body is also called the sensitive body or the soul. This body stores our feelings—our fears as well as our joys, instincts, prejudices, emotions, and impulses.

The mental body contains our ideas, beliefs, and perceptions of the experiences we have in life. What we normally call *mind* is pure activity. We cannot see it. We cannot treat it with surgery, as we can with the brain. It's the emerging phenomenon spreading out from the brain without limits, a *continuum* in and out of ourselves: inward through the PNIE network, inhabiting the body, and spreading outward beyond the body.[10] The brain is the *hardware,* and the mind is the *software.* Our mind continues outside our brain.

The Brain as an Antenna

For centuries, it was thought that the brain produces mental activity. But the mind as metaphor for the brain's program cannot explain spontaneity, creativity, or the fact that sometimes identical discoveries are made at the same time in different places in the world.

Recent studies in neuroscience show that the mind is also an antenna capturing ideas from outside, constantly receiving, processing, and providing information in the form of energy.[11] PNIE explains how the brain responds to our "perceptions" of what we are living, generates emotions, and sends orders to the immune system and the endocrine or hormonal system to regulate the internal environment and give an appropriate response to the experience. Thus, mental activity is not exclusively hosted in the brain.[12]

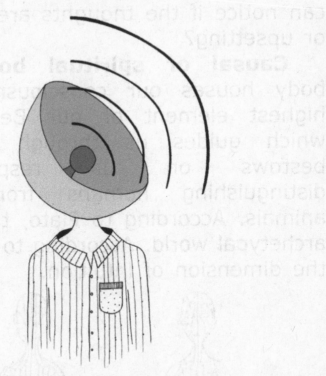

The brain as an antenna.

The words we speak are waves floating in space. We see this clearly in the 1997 sci-fi film *Contact,* in which scientists discern recognizable speech in the atmosphere, miles away from Earth.[13]

Our thoughts are energy and can be transmitted to others. Have you ever noticed how, when someone is concentrated, you can almost feel the thoughts in the air? And sometimes you can notice if the thoughts are pleasant or upsetting?

Causal or spiritual body: This body houses our consciousness, the highest element of our Being, that which guides us through life and bestows on us responsibility, distinguishing humans from other animals. According to Plato, this is the archetypal world. According to Jung, it's the dimension of intuition.

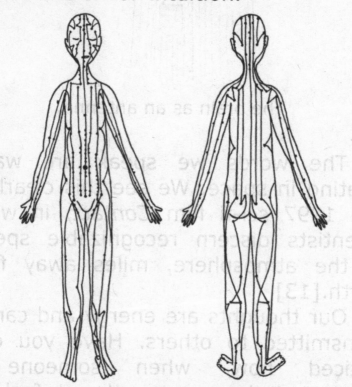

The meridian system.

Another way to describe our energetic body is through the meridians system of Chinese medicine. The human body has a system of energetic channels, called meridians, which connect all organs, tissues, and cells. The pathway of meridians is related to the pathways of the circulatory, nervous, and lymphatic systems. The vital energy circulating through the meridians is necessary to keep all organs and tissues active, to make them function properly, and to coordinate their activities.

Rocío continued to hold her hand on the pit of her stomach. I asked what was happening, and she said her stomach was in knots. "I've felt this way since my partner and I had an argument this morning. What can it be?" she asked.

I explained that it was the energy of the third chakra, located over the pit of the stomach. Through this chakra, we connect with others, and from this point we feel and hold emotions, like anger.

The word *chakra* comes from the Sanskrit word for wheel or disk. This ancient Indian religious language is based on understanding the spiritual nature of human beings. Chakras are energy centers. They have the form of a vortex, like a tornado spinning in both directions at the same time. We can sense them in the front and the back of our bodies. They are inside the vital or etheric body, in alignment with the spine. Though there are more, the best-known chakras are seven, numbered from the root chakra.

On the physical plane, a chakra is a torus,[14] a sphere continuously turning in on itself, a source of energy that pulses in an infinite feedback loop. Each chakra, or energy center, is activated with a certain color and a certain sound. And since light and sound produce geometrical figures, independent of any knowledge of sacred geometry, each energy center also has a particular form, as beautifully represented in Indian art.

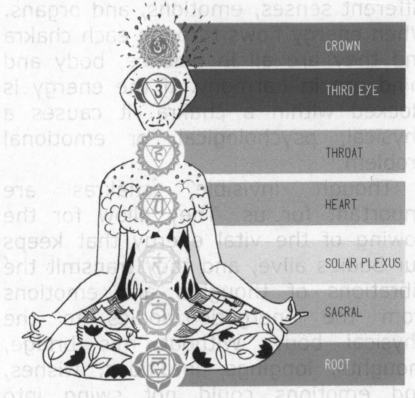

CROWN

THIRD EYE

THROAT

HEART

SOLAR PLEXUS

SACRAL

ROOT

The chakra system.

Chakras are living energy centers that act as an interface between our physical, emotional, mental, and spiritual bodies. Each chakra works as a transmitter and receiver of specific frequencies of energy. Together they function as an integrated system and are the primary means of our Soul's embodiment in physical form.[15]

Since the chakras rule the human energy system, they also regulate the different senses, emotions, and organs. When energy flows through each chakra and they are all in balance, body and mind are in harmony. If the energy is blocked within a chakra, it causes a physical, psychological, or emotional problem.

Though invisible, chakras are important for us. They allow for the flowing of the vital energy that keeps our bodies alive, and they transmit the vibrations of thoughts and emotions from the energetic bodies to the physical body. Without this bridge, thoughts, longings, intuitions, wishes, and emotions could not swing into action.

Like vortices, they absorb, transform, and distribute vital energy. The etheric or vital body captures the energy from the universe and from the environment (subtle energy from the sun, the earth, and the emotions) and sends it to the organs through the chakras. The chakras transform this subtle energy into energy that is assimilable by the body, and distribute it to the different organs.

Each chakra is bound to an endocrine gland that releases hormones into the bloodstream. Thus, the universe energy information reaches the body's cells through the hormones, connecting Heaven with Earth.

The first three chakras, which we share with the animal kingdom, regulate the basic functions of survival, sexuality, and eating. Human beings whose lives rely primarily on these chakras are those who find the meaning of their lives in power, sex, and success. They are individualistic and express themselves emotionally through fear, anger, suffering, longing, and anxiety.

The fourth and fifth chakras, typical of the human being, regulate how we give and receive love and how we show it.

The sixth and seventh chakras belong to the divine kingdom, where our most developed capacities are regulated. They are associated with intuition, intellect, imagination, knowledge, and spiritual longing. Persons who find their place on the four upper chakras are concerned with the common good, the evolution of human awareness, and making spiritual teachings conscious. They are governed by universal values like love, freedom, and equality, rather than by emotions.

Practice for Healthy Living

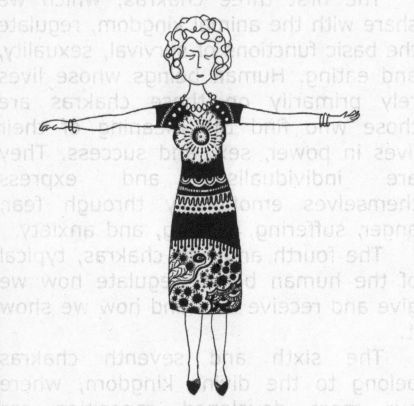

Healthy balance.

While standing or sitting, stretch your arms to the sides, like a weighing scale with its center in the heart chakra.

Your right hand gives and your left hand receives.

Close your eyes and allow your scale to weigh your sense of balance. What do you feel?

Which arm is heavier (giving or receiving)? Are you giving more than you are receiving, receiving more than giving, or do you feel balanced?

Our center fluctuates among the chakras, depending on the level of awakened consciousness in each moment.[16] (For more information on each chakra and its features, see appendix 3, "The Chakra System.")

Consciousness

Consciousness is the ability to know oneself and one's environment. It includes everything and enables us to awaken to multiple possibilities.

Living in a state of awakened consciousness, vibrating in the upper chakras, we enter into life fully, where the impossible becomes possible.

Chakras, like all organs of the body, function in a coordinated way, adjusting to one another. An unbalanced chakra affects the others' balance. When you need to regain physical and emotional harmony, it's important to balance the chakras.

Rocío and I finished our session by harmonizing the chakras through a sound meditation. She was able to relax and could feel the knots in her stomach disappear. For Rocío, it was a discovery to see how the energetic body functions. She'd found her fourth clue!

Rocío was interested in continuing to work with energy, and when she returned for our next consultation, she told me she had experienced a session of energy healing and that during the past few days she had felt calmer and less explosive.

We've all experienced strong emotions and seen how they prevent clear thought. Think of attending a sports event—the wave of feelings pushing you until you find yourself enraged, yelling, and sharing with people you've never seen before. The same happens when we fall in love; we feel a surge of inner strength and are emboldened to embark on new projects and adventures.

Practice for Healthy Living

How can I balance and cleanse my chakras?

There are exercises: physical exercises, breathing exercises, meditations, color and sound therapies, and crystal therapies to cleanse and balance the chakras.

How and what we eat also affects our chakras. Proteins nourish the root chakra. Liquids are best for the sacral chakra. Whole grains for the solar plexus chakra. Vegetables for the heart chakra. Fruits for the throat chakra. Each chakra will also be nourished by the fruits and vegetables with which it shares color vibrations. For example, the root chakra gets nourished from red fruits. The crown chakra is also nourished by fasting. A well-balanced diet nourishes the whole subtle body.

Attending a session of an energetic therapy designed to cleanse chakras can be useful. Having our chakras opened by another person is not always helpful, though. Sometimes chakras are out of alignment for a purpose. For example, when you are exposed to continuous aggression, it can be wise to close the solar plexus and heart chakras to protect yourself from a violent environment. As a temporary measure, this might be healthier than having all the chakras opened. If a therapist opens our chakras, we might return to an unhealthy situation vulnerable, so it's important to work with a therapist who is trained in alignment himself or herself and working in a conscious, responsible way, having the best intentions for our well-being.

Every action is preceded by an emotion, and each emotion is communicated instantaneously in a cascade of molecules that bring the information to all the cells in the body. When our feelings and thinking are in alignment, the emotion releases an energy that helps us navigate the world.

But when our emotions and mentation are out of synch, when we feel one thing and think another, we lack motivation and focus; and our creativity, problem-solving abilities, response time, and behavior are limited.

When we're stressed, we secrete cortisol, adrenaline, and other stress hormones that spread throughout the body, keeping us in alert mode. When we're happy, we release serotonin, which produces pleasant sensations. Each emotional state engenders a particular pattern of information molecules, which is why we can be taken by only one emotional state at a time. We can't be both angry and happy at the same time.

The Language of Emotions

Emotions are translated into molecules generated by the brain and the nervous networks that spread through the bloodstream and internal environment, sending information to different parts of the body. As they arrive at their destinations, these molecules activate receptors on the surface of the cells.

Body and mind form an indivisible whole, a network in which the information molecules function as messengers. Researchers used to think these molecules were secreted only by the nervous system, so they were called *neurotransmitters.* Recent research shows that some neurotransmitters are secreted to the bloodstream and act as hormones, so they are called *neurohormones.* Since neurotransmitters are formed by amino acids, they're also called *neuropeptides.* Candace Pert and her colleagues have shown how these neurotransmitters also deliver messages outside the nervous system. She calls them *molecules of emotion.* Considering that these molecules transmit information about emotions and other states of consciousness, we will refer to them as *information molecules.* The sum of these sixty or seventy molecules form the universal biochemical language of the emotions.

This is the language used in the PNIE network's communication system.

Practice for Healthy Living

Close your eyes.

Put your hand or hands on your heart.

Recall a moment when you received exceptionally good news.

Pay attention to your body.

Feel the wave of happiness molecules spreading inside you.

Recalling happy times is a treasure. It allows us to express our happiness biology, which positively affects our health.

Emotions bind our body and soul. They have an energetic, or spiritual, component that forms as feelings and sensations, and a physical component represented by information molecules and their receptors, binding both worlds. **Emotions are the great integrator of our being.**

We generally become aware of this only when there's a great wave of information molecules and we feel an emotion. In fact, there is a continuous, subtle waving of barely noticeable sensations and feelings. Thoughts and emotions sent by the mind are translated as **sensations and feelings** in the body. They are **the language used by the mind to talk through the body.**

Staying present with sensations and feelings is to enter the continuous flow of information that bathes our being in every moment. If you learn to listen to your mind-body, you'll be able to contact that information—the wisdom and intelligence of your body, the unconscious, preconscious, or subconscious. Neuroscientists use the term *nonconscious processes* to name all the activity carried out by consciousness that goes beyond the conscious mind, which includes the unconscious, the subconscious, etc. In this book, we refer to those nonconscious processes as *nonconscious mind,* to distinguish from the conscious mind.

Mind-body is a large field of fluctuating information. **You are not**

anchored to any moment. The dynamic balance, in movement, is a sign of health. In fact, the heart rate variability in a healthy person is chaotic and tends to follow a regular rhythm when we're ill or near death.

The Only Thing That's Permanent Is Change

Becoming aware of the mind speaking through the body, without words but with the language of sensations and feelings, allows us to bring more of our nonconscious mind to consciousness, illuminating our shadow. Yoga is a practice to accomplish this. *Yoga* means union, the union of mind and body as a whole.

Practices like Kum Nye (Tibetan yoga) are based on feeling as the clue to experience the mind-body union. While we are in contact with our mind-body, we can **align what we feel, think, and do and from there express our full potential.**

Feeling the Body Is Listening to the Mind Speaking a Nonverbal Language

Visualize mind-body as an iceberg. The portion above the surface is the *conscious mind,* the story I'm telling myself about what's happening. At this moment, you're conscious that you're reading this book.

Mind-Body

The relation between mind and body has been the subject of study among philosophers, yogis, and scientists for millennia.

There are basically two streams: Western dualist philosophy makes a rigid distinction between body and mind. The Eastern monistic view considers mind-body as an indivisible whole, a unit.

In the Western world, we have developed *conventional* medicine, which focuses on the body, and psychology and psychiatry, which deal with the mind. In the East, Chinese and Ayurvedic medicines consider mind-body as a whole.

The portion of the iceberg that's underwater is the *nonconscious mind.* There is considerably more nonconscious activity than conscious activity. Our mind hides a lot of vital information, both involuntary (autonomic) synchronization of bodily functions and those parts of our psyche that are suppressed and inaccessible (personal shadow and collective unconscious) that reveal themselves symbolically through dreams, images, sensations, and thoughts.

Practice for Healthy Living

Stop what you're doing.

Get into a comfortable position and close your eyes.

Focus inside, as though you can see, hear, smell, taste, and feel your inner self. Let yourself be surprised by the sensations and feelings. Follow one sensation and see if it moves, changes its intensity, moves to other places in the body.

> Then, using each breath as if it's a huge interior wave, join all the body's sensations.

Try to imagine what would happen if at this moment you were to take charge of your breathing, digesting what you've eaten, secreting hormones to maintain an internal balance, regulating your body temperature and pH, etc., performing all these activities while reading and processing the information in this book. Mission impossible! Luckily, there's a nonconscious mind responsible for the synchronization of these bodily functions. If we had to coordinate all this using our conscious mind, we would break down.

The nonconscious mind also allows us to perform other automatic activities like talking, walking, eating, and driving. When we drive for the first time, we use our conscious mind, but once driving becomes automatic, the nonconscious mind takes over.

If we listen to our nonconscious mind, it can provide relevant information to guide us through life. Research by

Dean Radin of the Institute of Noetic Sciences (www.noetics.org) shows how the body anticipates highly emotional future events and manifests physiological changes even before the conscious mind is aware of them. The information may appear in a dream or a sensation. A heavy or painful feeling, for example, is the body's way to tell us something's wrong. **A pleasant or light sensation, like happiness, tells us we're on the right path.**

Follow your bliss.[17]

Sometimes a part of us wants to be expressed, but we don't allow it; we suppress it. In an effort to emerge from our depths and express itself in consciousness, it might show up in the body, perhaps as a nuisance to get our attention, then as a pain that we might "cure" with medication, and finally as a disease. **A disease might be the soul making its voice heard.**

Quantum physics adds additional information about the mechanics the body-mind uses to express itself. The brain receives information from the body and compares it to past experiences—through memories and beliefs—and produces notions. These thoughts, attitudes, and beliefs produce energy and resonance patterns that accumulate in the body. These patterns also affect the cascade of information molecules.

Practice for Healthy Living

"First the body whispers, then it speaks, and finally it screams."

Try to see the ways your body-mind communicates with you.

When you feel concerned about something, where in your body do you feel it?

If you're feeling nervous because you have to give a speech or go to a difficult meeting, how does your body express it?

It's common to feel a concern as a headache and fear of public speaking as a knot in your stomach. However, your body-mind may communicate in some other way, and you may feel your concerns and stress elsewhere in your body.

> Each person is unique.
> Learn to understand the language through which your body talks to you.

When we become aware of how the resonance patterns produced by thoughts affect information molecules, we appreciate how our thoughts create the conditions of our body and our experiences. Understanding this, we can train the mind to produce thoughts that support our physical and emotional well-being—detach from problems and negative emotional states, live joyfully, and generate inner peace. **Training the mind to choose and sustain healthy thoughts is a full-time job.**

> Did you know that you can select your thoughts just as you select your clothes every day?[18]

Our thoughts frame the way we perceive and process the experiences we have and how we generate emotions. If we process our perceptions based on fear, we live as though under attack. If we see the world as abundant, we can be confident we'll get what we need.

Your Thoughts Determine the World You See[19]

Stimuli are always competing for our attention—sensations, memories, and thoughts. What you focus on becomes the framework of your world.

From the prefrontal cortex, the part of the brain behind the forehead that distinguishes us from other higher mammals and makes us human, we can select what we want to pay attention to at every moment.

If we pay attention primarily to injustice, what we see will be filtered through the lens of injustice, which will shape our construction of facts. Someone with a different filter will see another reality, even if the facts are the same.

We organize the data we receive *from the inside.* When we look through rose-colored glasses, we see the world in rose. We construct what happens to us through our choice of where we place our attention and our frame of reference.

The future is not cast in stone. We "create" it with our thoughts, emotions, and decisions. Any "muscle" we exercise becomes stronger and leaves a well-worn path, which grooves into a pattern that defines the way we'll experience similar situations in the future. **We create our own reality.**

Emotions have been preserved through evolution because they are useful for survival. In some way, they are protective. An emotion in itself is neither good nor bad. Like fire, if we use it for cooking it's beneficial; if it rages out of control it's problematic. Whether fire is good or bad, beneficial or problematic, depends on how we use it.

Anger helps us become aware of the volcano we have deep inside. The same happens when we are filled with joy. These different moments help us to be aware of all the energy we have within ourselves.

Where does all this energy go? It's often said that energy flows where attention goes. Our thoughts manage the energy. Poorly managed energy can be harmful. If we think about a problem all day long, it will tend to increase. If energy follows attention, our thoughts matter!

Can Thoughts and Emotions Make Us Sick?

Just as our thoughts and emotions change from moment to moment, so does the PNIE network. All our cells have receptors for information molecules, so our moods are reflected instantaneously in our immune system.

White blood cells are bits of the brain floating around the body. I'm not able to differentiate clearly the brain from the rest of the body.

—Candace Pert

From her research, Candace Pert, a pioneer in the field of psycho-neuro-immuno-endocrinology and other areas, posits that the immune system, including the central nervous system, has memory and the capacity to learn.

Thus, we can say that intelligence is located in every cell and distributed throughout the body, that the separation of psyche and soma, mind and body, is no longer a valid distinction. Pert explains that her study of receptors present in nerve cell membranes led her to discover that these same "neural" receptors are present in most, if not all, the body's cells.

Our thoughts and beliefs, and our perceptions of the experiences we have, give rise to emotions that express themselves internally through the PNIE system, producing information molecules that affect our internal environment. If we perceive a stressor, the alert mode is activated and stress molecules are released. When this happens on a chronic basis, stress molecules will depress the immune system, making it more vulnerable to illness.[20]

In this paradigm, **thoughts and emotions affect the body** and make us—more or less—vulnerable to illness. This helps explain how a chronic emotional imbalance can promote the onset of a new cancer and sustain the *cancering* mode.

We have already seen in chapter 3, "Why Do We Get Sick?" that getting sick has to do with the interaction of multiple chronic factors, including environmental pollution, poor eating habits, sedentary lifestyle, ineffective stress management, and negative emotional states. **Just one factor at only one time does not produce cancer.** A single negative thought or a single violent emotion is not by itself the cause of a disease, nor is a single instance of binge eating. Recurring negative thoughts, however, can give rise to repetitive patterns of information molecules that make the body vulnerable to disease.

If we bring our attention to our own care, to what fills our heart, to what is really important for us, the energy of our emotions will be motivated toward healthy habits. If we give emotions meaning as messengers and redirect their powerful energies, we'll be inclined to live a healthier life.

Human relationships are the ideal platform to generate emotions. In order to be accepted socially, it is common to hide our negative emotions such as anger, jealousy, or an overbearing eagerness to get something, the traits that agitate us and cause ourselves and others to suffer. But when we repress our emotions, they remain beneath our conscious awareness, and when they're triggered, we blame others—society, the lack of money—for our suffering. We expend a lot of energy keeping the lid on this pressure cooker inside us.

The Body Accumulates an Influx of Negative Emotions

It's advisable to practice a regular cleanse of accumulated emotions (see chapter 9, "Tuning Up") in the same way we brush our teeth daily.

Rocío's inner work, trying to know more about herself, to nourish and balance her energetic body, was proceeding well. She realized how easily she got angry, and something was beginning to change inside her. She was able to identify situations that in the past might have resulted in explosive anger but that now she was able to react to in a different way. She could express what she was feeling and set clear limits to unhealthy situations. She continued moving forward through her treasure hunt, shining light on more and more aspects of herself.

During our next consultation, Rocío told me about a family scene that had taken place recently. It was her niece's birthday party, and her parents kept giving her orders—stop eating so much, stay out of the sun, dress warmly, stop running around with her nephews. "In the past, I would have lost it and screamed, 'Stop!' But this time I took ten conscious breaths and explained to them that I'm not a girl any longer and they can rely on me to make my own decisions." When she left, her aunts commented that she was calmer and brighter than they'd seen before. Her aunts' comments confirmed to Rocío that her changes were becoming noticeable.

We can't always change our circumstance, but we have a choice about how we'll respond. We can see the body-mind as purely material and static, or as an expression of consciousness. If we choose the latter, we open ourselves to the mystery of multiple possibilities. In every moment, **the mind-body uses different languages to express to us an underlying, unified field of consciousness.**

The Body Is Bubbling with Intelligence[21]

The body-mind is filled with intelligence. And that intelligence is located not just in the brain, but in every cell of your body.

Sometimes you feel there's "something you cannot digest." The brain might express this through brooding thoughts. The abdomen expresses it as a knot in the stomach.

Each cell of the body is conscious and expresses happiness, anguish, and anger in its own way and communicates it to the other cells.

Emotional states are states of consciousness. We go from one state of consciousness to another; and each is related to a typical wave of information molecules, sensed as particular emotions and producing certain physical effects, specific gestures, and behaviors. Whenever a consciousness pattern is activated in us, we act out the collective memories and behaviors imprinted by that pattern. As we've seen before, when we're at a football game we feel overtaken by a dominant emotion and act as puppets, dancing choreographed football-fan behaviors, even if we've never been to a game before.

This is clearly seen in individuals with multiple personality disorder or dissociative identity disorder. Under a given personality, they suffer from a disease, which then disappears when they identify with another personality. A person who suffers from diabetes and needs treatment, upon a change of personality, doesn't need the medication anymore. Another person needs corrective lenses for one personality, but not for the other.

> *Our bodies are more like a flickering flame than a hunk of meat.*
> —Candace Pert

These disorders confirm that we're like flickering flames, constantly changing. To think of ourselves as fixed is illusory. The body changes, depending on which consciousness is inhabiting it. **Consciousness creates reality.**

Thus, we have the choice to change from one emotional state to another and from one physical state to another. We live a realm of multiple potentials, and **this versatility lasts throughout our lives.**[22] The range of possible expressions in us is more powerful than any drug and makes us responsible for our own emotions and thoughts. We can train our mind to create a wholesome, healthy reality.

These sessions focusing on self-knowledge gave Rocío a broader view of who she is, and she became aware of new ways of self-perception, acknowledging that her identification with the thoughts "I am explosive" and "I am what I am" was no longer valid.

She had found her great treasure: a being bubbling with intelligence and multiple possibilities of expression. Repeating the same story about who she is had become unnecessary. She could choose her best self.

Rocío celebrated finding her vast possibilities, a treasured milestone on her path. Looking out at the horizon, she left my office wondering: "So, who am I?"

Neuro- and PNIE-Plasticity

We've seen in chapter 5, "Energize Your Body!," how dynamic the brain is. With its neuroplasticity, it can adapt according to the person's environment, psyche, and actions.

University of London researchers showed that the hippocampus, the area of the brain associated with spatial memory, is significantly bigger in London taxi drivers than in others. By memorizing the city's streets, these cabdrivers stimulated the development of that area of the brain. This did not diminish, but actually improved with years.

Neuroplasticity is the ability of the brain to form new neural connections *throughout life.* The brain changes form according to the areas used most, correlated with the mental activity. **By training our mind, we mold our brain structure.**

Like the nervous system, the PNIE network also has the ability to generate new circuits and adapt existing ones, affecting the secreting patterns of information molecules.

Neuro- and PNIE-plasticity allow for changing habits, conduct adjustment, and molding our mind-body throughout life. All of us have this treasure. Let's enjoy it!

Take-Home Message

We are not anchored or fixed to anything: Our body-mind is constantly reshaping itself.

Sensations, feelings, and emotions are the language the mind uses to speak through the body.

Feelings and emotions affect the body and can make us sick.

Our plasticity lasts throughout our lives.

***

Training our mind daily allows us to create a healthy reality.

Tracking pleasant sensations keeps us on a healthy path.

Aligning feeling, thinking, and doing is a clue to express our potential.

Dancing with the flow of life brings our body health and joy.

Chapter 8

DO I KNOW WHO I AM?

The most important kind of freedom is to be what you really are.

—JIM MORRISON

When Lorena, managing director of a multinational company, came to my office, she had a history of uterine cancer. She was receiving anticancer treatments and wanted to know whether there was anything else she could do to prevent recurrence. We talked about an integrative approach—the importance of making lifestyle changes and stimulating her immune system. After exploring her situation, we found that family relationships were bringing her out of balance.

After several sessions, she came in one day shaken by an argument she'd had with her partner. First, her grouchy side had come up; then a few minutes *later, she found herself in the arms of her partner, feeling like a little girl just wanting to be cuddled. "If I can change from being a monster into a vulnerable little girl in just a few minutes," she asked, "when I say 'I,' who am I talking about?"*

A good question! **As we grow, we continuously create our own personality.** Our personality isn't something we're born with. We continuously forge it.

The word *personality* comes from the Latin *persona*, referring to actors' masks in the theaters of old. What we call personality is a complex amalgam of sensations, thoughts, behaviors, fears, and emotions.

As we have to face difficult or painful situations, we behave in certain ways to protect ourselves, to protect our most vulnerable side. Personality is a pattern of attitudes, thoughts, feelings, and behaviors adopted and repeated, which come to characterize a person. These patterns tend to be stable and persistent throughout life, allowing us to predict how that person will act. If as a child, for example, our brothers taunted us for crying, we might choose to hide our crying or to attack and chase them away. If the latter strategy works, from then on when facing difficult or threatening situations, we might resort to aggression to protect the crying child.

Like actors, we employ more than one mask. Our personality has multiple sub-actors. Depending on the circumstance, we engage the actor who can cope best with the situation at hand: the brave self or the wise self or the receptive self. We all have within us similar sub-personalities, but you won't necessarily use the same one as someone else in the same situation. This distinguishes one person from another. The ego's sub-nature takes control of the situation and reacts in accord with its calculations, expectations, and evaluation of the previous mission.

What we call *self* might be the ego identified with a particular sub-actor, but the self is much more than that. If we identify with one sub-actor, we miss the chance to explore the depth and breadth of who we are.

How Many Are We, Actually, When We Think We Are Only One?[1]

As the artist and filmmaker Alejandro Jodorowsky said, "Ordinary people ... do not develop their human abilities, but live locked up in something they call *self.* It is as if they live only in one room of a huge mansion! So ordinary people make only one thing in their lives, and that is to use a label."[2]

What we call *personality* is a theater troupe, a bevy of sub-actors living inside us who go on stage when directed to do so by the ego. All these sub-actors, even those not on stage, are present as the inner voices we hear in continuous dialogue within our mind—and not under our control.

How Can Astrology Help Us on the Path of Self-Awareness?

Astrology is an ancient practice based on a holistic view of the human being and the universe. There are many ways to study and apply it.

Using the natal, or birth, chart to display who we are, astrology offers an invitation to conceive ourselves as a point of consciousness reflecting the world. Each of us, more or less, reflects all signs and planets, but in any given moment, we identify more with some than others. Our charts allow us to discover the players that are part of our troupe.

At any given time, a warrior or a conqueror might show up at work, while a tender, affectionate being remains hidden from our colleagues and appears only in intimate settings. Likewise, there are other characters who form parts of ourselves that we've not yet identified.

Through a holistic reading of our chart, we can recognize the characters who are a part of ourselves—those with whom we identify and those with whom we don't. The dynamic, fluid, and harmonious articulation of all these characters allows us to live more fully and faithfully to the fullness of our being.

Recognizing repressed or repudiated characters can lead to attitudes, practices, and decisions that shine light on the unconscious parts of ourselves. If, for example, we discover through our chart that we have a highly creative side, recognizing it and putting it into action through artistic activity can help us live more fully.

I explained to Lorena that when we say *self*, we're generally referring to the ego as stage director, the one responsible for deciding which sub-actor of our personality will show up. This is the self that most people identify with, the one Western society values. This is the *lower self*, as opposed to the *middle self* and *higher self*, which are related to our soul and spirit.

Lorena had been having problems at work. Her staff was calling her a despot. During the next session, we concentrated on analyzing her astrological chart, allowing her to identify and trace the origin of her bossy character. "I'm the oldest of five. When each of my brothers were born, my mother asked me to help take care of them. I no longer had time to draw, which had been my favorite activity. So I became my brothers' boss. I took on the same role at school and college, and now at work. Am I really bossy?"

Lorena and I continued our discussion about personality, which is constantly forming and re-forming as we grow. It is the mask we create to protect us. As if we were clay dolls, we're shaped by the experiences we have and the rules from the outside that condition our lives. If a response or role turns out to be useful, we'll probably use it again in similar situations. I used the example of a boy being picked on by his classmates. If he responds aggressively, shouting and cursing and threatening to fight, and sees that the other boys flee and do not bother him again, he's likely to employ an aggressive response in the future when he feels fear. That's how we adopt patterns, directing different characters onstage for different circumstances.

The ego is an energy structure that organizes different aspects of our personality, helping us function in the world, interacting and coping with the experiences we get. A healthy ego is our project manager, the organizer of our sub-personalities.

The ego is, thus, a tool. It was created to provide assistance to our lower self, not the other way around. Its function is to serve as director. But sometimes when our ego orders one sub-actor to go on stage more often than the other sub-actors, the ego begins to *identify with* it. It loses touch with the range of sub-actors in the troupe and loses its effectiveness as director. Although the others remain under its authority, the ego that doubles as principal actor is unhealthy. The play of life remains incomplete, the other players remain unfulfilled, and life loses its meaning.

In the case of Lorena, having had to assume an adult role as a child, responsible for her brothers' well-being, she left aside her creative, free, and playful side and had been onstage instead in a bossy and despotic role. She also felt like a boss in the rest of her life, clearly in identification with this sub-actor, the boss, and not able to express the full array of who she actually is.

The mind does not distinguish between what's actually happening and what we're imagining. When you imagine a delicious meal, the brain thinks you're sitting in front of the food, and the mouth salivates, preparing for digestion. The ego creates situations in the mind—imaginary productions that unleash a chain of thoughts, energy, and emotions, as though they were actually happening. The ego is an *energy structure* and nourishes itself from energy. It feeds itself from emotions it creates.

The Aim of an Unhealthy Ego Is Survival

The ego helps us function as individuals. Unfortunately, this can be accomplished in a way that makes us feel isolated rather than connected with others. An egoist, someone who is arrogant, makes one sub-character in the troupe of actors the principal and identifies with it, rather than serving as director of the whole company.

The survival instinct is an extremely powerful force within us. Under duress, people accomplish superhuman feats, like swimming great distances or overturning heavy objects.

When the ego functions from the survival instinct, it doesn't care about who or what is left behind. The only issue is survival at all costs. When the ego takes the lead in this way, there isn't room for spirit.

Whenever the ego identifies with a certain sub-actor, it will create emotions that nourish only this sub-actor. The emotions will reinforce this sub-actor, and as the sub-actor's role increases, the ego will give it even more airtime and a wider range of emotions, even allowing it to manage its thoughts and feelings.

Lorena and I did some exercises to help her recognize the conversations that take place in her mind. "The people I supervise at work are useless! If I don't tell them exactly what to do, they don't do anything!"

Practice for Healthy Living

Take moments of silence and peacefulness throughout the day to touch your own essence. Stillness brings peace.

During the following sessions, Lorena and I explored her recurring thoughts. Slowly, she began to realize that her own inner dialogue created the anger that made her want to "kick everyone out." This feeling made her "boss" more and more inflated, reinforcing the idea that "the only way anything can happen is to make everyone work harder, continuously raising the goalposts for her staff." And the anger kept feeding itself and confirming the necessity of having a strong "boss."

She began to understand that reality isn't as bad as she imagined. If she allowed her staff to act independently, she'd be surprised by the ideas they generated. She understood how her projections affected her perceptions, continuously feeding the "boss" and making it more dominant.

Practice for Healthy Living

Find a calm place, close your eyes, and look inward. What situations do you imagine? Are you the victim, the perpetrator, or the rescuer? Do you have recurring thoughts that make you think you're right, the best? Or do you feel helpless?

Try to see which sub-actor you identify with. Tell your ego you are much more than one sub-actor and you need to let others go onstage, too.

Let your spirit guide you with wisdom and love.

Write all that you notice in your journal.

Look at your ego and recognize when it's taking over, not acting as a director but as the main actor. Awareness is the first step to disidentify from the mask the ego has imposed on us and will allow us to uncover our real selves and realize our potential.

"There is nothing more important in the path of personal growth than realizing that we are not the voice in our brain, but the person who is listening to it."[3] We create the voices inside us to protect ourselves. Our essence, which is always paying attention and is aware of the chatter, is quiet.

Ego isn't a bad thing. It has a protective function, choosing the characters that help us face life's challenges. When we identify with a defiant or aggressive character, our ego gives us the courage and power we need. But perhaps we don't need it as frequently now and decide to set it aside for special occasions.

> *My soul is a secret orchestra; but I don't know what instruments—strings, harps, cymbals drums—strum and bang inside me. I only know myself as the symphony.*
> —Fernando Pessoa, *The Book of Disquiet*[4]

Once we're able to recognize our identification with a certain character, it's important to express our gratitude for helping us become what we are today, honoring the journey that brought us here. But when the journey has taken us away from who we actually are, it's time to return to ourselves. The aim isn't to stop being the person we've been, but to realize we are much more than that. It's not a matter of silencing the principal actor, but including many others in the troupe as well. We're much more than one character, and it's time to include all our different parts.

Lorena agreed that her character as a boss had served her well, not only at home helping her overburdened mother, but in subsequent situations, too. In her current work for a multinational corporation, she was entrusted with a large team whose members were pretty much her age, and yet she had to be the boss. She was thankful for her "boss" character, who came onstage and helped her take this responsibility. Now she realized she'd been mistaken to take that role in all situations. Doing so was making her suffer.

Becoming aware that we're not *only* the character we thought we were can be a difficult awakening. It's advisable to traverse this path with a highly experienced therapist. Realizing that we're not actually our first or last names, our neighborhood, our home, the family vacations that gave us our identity can shake our world, make us feel unstable, even terrify us. But it's also liberating to discover the many other characters within us, to reset ourselves and align more faithfully with who we actually are.

Lorena was enthusiastic about what she was discovering. I suggested she take painting classes to contact her other characters, and she discovered the creativity she had abandoned years ago.

Lorena wanted to explore what had caused her to be the way she was. She had a three-year-old daughter and a one-year-old son. She didn't want to repeat her patterns with them. "Above all, I want my daughter to enjoy being

a little girl, something I could not do,"
she told me.

I explained to Lorena how we're conditioned from a young age to act certain ways. Even grade school students have impossibly tight schedules plus after-school activities like piano lessons, dance, and sports. Parents become a taxi service, which adds stress to their days over and above their own work hours.

As adults, we feel the pressure of time, the obligation to *do,* to fulfill the myriad duties we impose on ourselves, to be like others, to feel like we really belong. Life passes by while we live by our schedules and to-do lists, and the day comes when we realize we forgot to be alive.[5] Many people today feel that their lives are out of control. It's as if they only breathe during weekends and holidays.

Conditioned rules ("shoulds") have been adopted by us and become habits—somatic and neural pathways we don't even realize we're following. We act automatically, without awareness. After following these pathways so many times, we cannot step out of these grooves. As we saw in chapter 7, "The Treasure Hunt," it's wired into our nervous system by neurons connecting among themselves. If we activate the same neural circuitry repeatedly, it becomes automatic.

This patterning also leaves its mark on our energetic body. Repeated experiences gradually become installed in our vital body and modify pre-existing molds and patterns. In this way, new grooves are created that function as new rules conditioning behavior. The new patterns form molds for the postures and attitudes of the physical body. As long as we walk the same grooves again and again, we can't break our habits.

Reactions are attitudes and emotions that are triggered automatically in response to certain stimuli. It's as if someone presses a button and our pre-programmed reaction comes up. Becoming conscious means to be present and open to what's actually happening, to the stimuli and the urges to respond habitually, and to respond instead according to current needs, without being constricted by past actions.

Practice for Healthy Living

Whenever a negative emotion arises, stop.

Breathe slowly, and count each breath, from one to ten.

Doing this is a way to turn off automatic pilot.

Take the reins of your life and find the best response to each situation.

Our preprogrammed response, our habitual lead character, was useful during a certain period of our life, but when it becomes useless or even interferes with presence and the ways we relate to others, it's time to return to the drawing board. Trying to discern the reaction patterns we fall into nonconsciously is the beginning of mindful awareness and the ability to modify them.

Body-mind is a complete whole. Working with the body-mind allows us to change patterns more easily. With conscious body work, we relax our structures and loosen some of the conditioned patterns that have been established in our energetic body. We untie knots and open new circuits. Neuroplasticity allows us to modify neuronal pathways and turn nonconscious reactions into fresh responses. In the same way that we established unhealthy behavioral patterns, we can struggle back along the same path and create healthy patterns.

Lorena and I talked about all this. She was learning about her own conditioning patterns and could use these insights raising and educating her children.

Buddhism teaches that we are like seeds. If we're constrained by conditioning, the seeds might not be able to grow. Our being, our essence, remains latent until conditions are favorable for germination. Then we can blossom. When the time is right, our soul will offer clues, e.g., a feeling of dissatisfaction at work that might grow into a general dissatisfaction with life. "I've struggled to build a family, get promotions at work, yet in my heart I know that something is missing. I'm not happy." These are calls of the soul encouraging us to attend to our inner life and become the person we truly are.

I made it clear to Lorena that the fate of her children was not only dependent on how she raised them. We're all members of the same family, even before birth. If one person has a problem, everyone is affected. Psychogenealogy, a new discipline arising from psychotherapy, sees the family as a systemic body with ongoing relationships. From this point of view and on the basis of complex systems theory, if one person has a problem, we're all affected by it. We carry our complete family tree with us. Psychogenealogy explains, for example, how a family's secrets affect all its members and how what is silenced in one generation can appear in the body of later generations. In this way, an illness can be an invitation to explore a conflict in our family tree. Living consciously gives us the opportunity to solve conflicts for the whole family.

Lorena understood that although her role was not the only factor affecting her children's development, she did feel responsible for creating conditions that respected her children's leisure and creativity times, to allow their seeds to germinate as they grew up.

It was satisfying to see Lorena start to live more consciously and apply what she was learning to her family, becoming an exemplary mom. If we were all raised that consciously, there would be far less evil, violence, and illness in the world.

At our next session, Lorena wanted to share a dream. "I'm huge, as though a giant, and I'm talking with a normal-sized version of myself. The giant knows all my secrets. It comforts me, indicating that I'm on the right track. I can still see the image of a long path in front of me."

"Who is this giant talking to me with such wisdom?" she asked. To respond, I introduced the three levels of self.

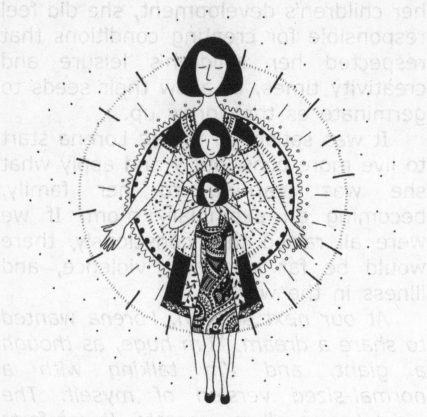

The three levels of the self.

What is usually called *self,* the self to which we've been referring, can be called the *lower self,* consisting of our ego and personality. This self is connected to the first three chakras, particularly the third: the solar plexus. Most people identify with this self—the ones whose demands and values contemporary society is designed to satisfy.

The soul can be called the *middle self.* It's related to the fourth and fifth chakras—our capacity to love and express what we feel—and serves as a bridge between the lower self and the higher self, or spirit.

We usually visualize the *higher self,* or *spirit,* as beyond our body, a giant, but it's also a part of ourselves. It is related to the sixth and seventh chakras, particularly the seventh. The spirit or higher self is the wisdom and love that supports our soul. If the soul is a drop of water in the ocean, spirit is the whole ocean.

Have You Ever Felt You Were One with Others?

A choir, group dancing, spiritual practices within a community—all of these give us a taste of being a drop of water in the vast ocean.

Most important is to align the three levels of self. The ego helps us live well day-to-day when we employ it in harmony with soul and spirit. But if we identify only with our lower self and our ego, we'll be controlled by hatred, sin, ambition, envy, and jealousy. We'll live contracted and confined to our lower self. We can feel this in our third chakra: our abdomen.

The soul allows us to connect with what is important in life. If we cultivate soul, our heart will open, and we'll be eager to share our feelings—to embrace and be embraced. We'll live a more affectionate life, harmonious and in service to others. We'll be self-confident and live without fear.

The spirit or higher self is our essence, the wisest part of ourselves. Spirit leads ego. When ego is in accord with spirit, we know how to get along in the world. We won't be egocentric; we'll be empathic, feeling what happens to others. Unlike ego, spirit helps us feel connected, a part of the larger whole. Connected with spirit, we realize that separateness is an illusion.

Practice for Healthy Living

The eyes are the door to the soul.

When was the last time you looked someone in the eyes?

Make eye contact, without using words, only gazing from soul to soul with another.

Record your feelings.

You may be moved to conclude with a loving embrace, from heart to heart.

Through spiritual practices leading to self-knowledge, we can increase our energy level and cultivate the superior self, be open to it, and be able to sustain its presence in our life. Spirit guides us, gives us advice in the form of insights, and leads us through our life. When we're walking our path and fulfilling our purpose, we live with wisdom, love, peace, and confidence.

Illness can show us that we're diverging from our path, that ego has taken the driver's seat and isn't in alignment with soul. "The body drains the soul's message." Cancer forces us to stop and look at how we are living. It invites us to reconnect with spirit and get back on a healthy course, consistent with our life's purpose.

It seemed Lorena's soul had visited in her dreams, coming to assure her she was back on track and encouraging her to continue. She recognized that in her dream, for the soul had reconnected her with spirit. She learned a lot from one dream. I advised her to record her dreams in her journal.

> *Illness is the result of a conflict between the purposes of the soul and the personality's actions and outlook.*
> —Dr. Edward Bach

Doctor as Guide

Looking at a person *as a whole,* their unfolding, clarifies how they have come to this point and how to help them understand their situation in a larger context.

To help a person's ego regain its role as director, I have to align with the soul. My intention is to guide individuals from identification with the individual self, which is mortal, to the collective self. When reunited with all beings, our essence resonates and we step into eternity.

Lorena was moving forward at a staggering speed. She knew herself increasingly well. One day she brought to our session an issue she was having. When she was with friends with whom she felt at ease, she could speak her mind and share her heart freely. But when her friend Paula was present, Lorena felt harassed and insecure and could hardly speak about what she was experiencing.

Our encounters with others nourish us and feed our relationships. As social beings, we discover ourselves and our ideas in response to what we see in others. We project what is unknowable in us onto another, who functions as a mirror, reflecting back what we are unable to see in ourselves. In this way, we interweave with others our own personality, intermingling our lives. It works both ways. We are a mirror for them as well. Although most of this takes place nonconsciously, we both have the opportunity to learn about ourselves, to see places that are hard to see. We learn a lot about others by seeing who they spend time with, because others hold characteristics we rarely express (and are probably nonconscious) but are very much a part of us.

Making projections conscious, taking off blinders, is not a bed of roses. It's difficult to walk the path of self-knowing. "The other person adds what's lacking in my own life, the things I can't see or don't pay attention to."[6]

Lorena continued diving deeply. What was she projecting onto Paula that was so inhibiting? What did Paula remind her of? When in her life had she felt this insecure?

We behave differently depending on who's around. We choose which part of ourselves to show, how to behave, with whom to identify. Who is present determines, in part, who we are in that moment, and so we can say they are a part of us.

Are you always the same person when you're with one of

your parents, with a friend, or with someone who works with you?

When in the presence of an authority, we might show a more dependent side of ourselves. When we're with friends or colleagues with whom we feel comfortable, we might exhibit more independence and be more daring. An authoritarian personality tends to be obedient, but when the same person cultivates real friendships, freedom and creativity can develop.

We're affected by whom we're with. You might have thought that when two people meet, each comes with his own personality and together they create a unique relationship. One plus one equals two. Rather than two independent people meeting at a point, each person emerges as a result of their interaction: two is equal to one plus one.

Thus, our self is formed gradually as we create new relations, first with our family, then in school, and as we grow up, with every relationship. All our contacts, pleasant and unpleasant, leave a trace. **Who you relate to and how you relate are important.**

Lorena was able to see how she showed different parts of herself depending on who was present. She became aware that in the presence of Paula, it was the insecure Lorena who had appeared when as a child there were unknown people in her home. Shy Lorena reappeared in her relationship with Paula.

In chapter 7, "The Treasure Hunt," we saw how we're a physical body, extended by an energetic body—where thoughts, emotions, and feelings flow, and extended further in a *continuum* with our relationships. We're like fish in the sea. When a distant fish moves, we feel the pulse in the water, even if we never touch each other.

Practice for Healthy Living

Have you ever felt, when entering a room, a good or bad "vibe"?

Have you ever been in the presence of someone emitting calmness and peace, and you feel fine just being there?

Invite a friend or family member to share an experience with you. Close your eyes and ask your friend or relative to move closer to you slowly and quietly. Can you feel when this person entering your sphere of influence, touching your energetic body?

In the same way, we constantly affect each other with our thoughts and emotions, even when we don't express them aloud. **We think we're separate, but that's an illusion.** With this in mind, **start by cultivating peace within.**

"To love our neighbor as ourselves"[7] requires that we love ourselves first. When we're in alignment, balanced, and flowing, we're able to transmit these feelings to those we meet and to tune in to the frequency of those qualities in them, whether we talk to each other or not. Even in line in the supermarket, we're influencing those around us, positively or negatively. **The trace we leave on the world is our responsibility.**

Take-Home Message

Our personality is forged as we mature.

Dis-identifying from solely our personality allows us to align with our soul and spirit.

Spiritual practices help us feel healthy within and connected to the world and all other people.

We influence each other, either positively or negatively. It's important to choose whom we relate to, and how.

The trace we leave on the world is our responsibility.

Chapter 9

TUNING UP

Freedom lies in being bold.
                              —ROBERT FROST

Yanina, a thirty-nine-year-old woman with a three-year-old daughter, was undergoing chemo to reduce the size of a breast tumor so that it could be removed surgically. Her friend told her about integrative medicine. When we met, I offered Yanina the image of a vegetable garden and the need for ongoing tending so the plants would stay healthy and thrive. "I understand, Laura," she said, "but won't I be fine after they remove the tumor? I'm so tired; I just want my life back."

I agreed that removing the tumor was most important but added that surgery wasn't all she needed. The tiredness she was feeling showed that her body needed revitalization—renewed energy—to help her recovery.

When we feel we lack energy, it's literally true. Energy that is expended needs to be regenerated. The energetic body gives us warnings—we feel tired; we think we're hungry; we might have a pain or the feeling of heaviness. When we ignore these warnings and go on and on without replenishing our energy, the body has to work too hard. If the situation stays the same, we start to get sick.

The vital body provides the energy that mobilizes the physical body, so our vital energy needs constant renewal. As noted in chapter 5, "Energize Your Body!," we restore our energy by means of a healthy diet, sound sleep, breathing exercises, meditation and other anti-stress techniques, and devoting time to activities and people that we enjoy.

I asked Yanina about her life, trying to understand why she was so tired. "These last years have been difficult. I work ten or twelve hours a day in a factory, with a lot of responsibility and stress, and this year there have been serious problems at work. In addition, I've been taking care of my mother, who was battling breast cancer. When she died, I thought I'd be more relaxed, but then I was diagnosed with cancer."

Yanina's life was one of long work hours and family demands, raising a young daughter and caring for her ailing mother. Worrying whether her mother would respond to treatment or not was an added stress, on top of the time and energy spent taking care of her. With these stressors taking her attention, she hadn't noticed her tumor until it was at an advanced stage.

I told Yanina that her busy lifestyle had led to a severe imbalance. The long-term stress had affected her PNIE network, and this system's failure had created a field conducive to cancer developing. As with computer hard disks when they're full, we need to stop from time to time to delete what's no longer needed and be able to reconnect with ourselves.

How can an imbalance in the energetic body produce an illness? Agitation, emotional demands, and loss of meaning or purpose affect our energetic body and produce an imbalance in our mental, emotional, and spiritual bodies, adversely affecting the physical body.

We know that **our beliefs and thoughts generated in our mental body affect our physical body** due to their direct connection with the brain. When we assign negative meaning to our experiences based on fear or abusive thoughts, an imbalance is created in the **mental body,** which affects the representations or images in the brain. Mental images are translated into information molecules through the PNIE network. In the body, negative images are translated into stress molecules or negative emotions.

In the same way, emotions affect the chakras that, through their connections with specific glands and surrounding organs, affect different parts of the physical body. Any emotion dammed up in the **emotional body** produces a disruption in a chakra, which will affect the part of the body that chakra is connected with and, through the production of hormones, will affect the rest of the body. When one chakra is not in balance with the other chakras, this brings about hormonal disturbances and disturbances of the PNIE network, also affecting the immune system.

The loss of values and meaning reflect a disconnection from our **spiritual body,** which leads us to identify with ego, thus producing an imbalance in our being. This is how a spiritual disconnect can be a cause of illness.

If an imbalance in our energetic body persists over time, it will be felt as a disturbance at the physical level and produce what we call *disease*. It's important to pay attention to all dimensions of our humanness to maintain or recover good health.[1]

Different Medicines for Different Dimensions of Our Being

Medicine deals primarily with disturbances of the physical body.

Psychology focuses on movements in the emotional and mental dimensions.

A healer focuses on the energetic body and its impact on the physical body.

> Holistic medical systems, e.g., anthroposophy or Chinese and Ayurvedic medicine, are based on maintaining health or balance in all of our being (between the physical and energetic bodies).

I strongly supported Yanina pursuing "conventional" anticancer treatment, but told her how important it is to also pay attention to all parts of herself, especially in light of the stresses and disruptions of the past year. Conventional medicine heals only the body, and does not yet pay much attention to stress, one of the most frequent causes of illness today. Illness affects more than one level, and if all levels aren't treated, the illness might appear again. If someone gets sick due to emotional blockage, for example, even when the physical illness is treated, it might recur or the person might develop another illness related to the same blockage.

This is why it's important **to become aware of our energetic body** and introduce practices into our daily life to keep the body in balance. These practices should include **a cleanse of accumulated and recurrent emotions or thoughts** to let the energy flow freely within the system. We all have the power to transform ourselves, to harmonize our energetic body, and keep ourselves strong and in balance. No pill can do this.

The Body as a Musical Instrument

Each chakra is a musical note. If we are in tune, we'll be able to express our melody, the sound of our true self.

Thoughts, emotions, wishes, and intuitions all reverberate through the physical body. If they aren't in accord with who we really are, the sounds will be dissonant.

Many therapies use sounds, based upon the legacy of Pythagoras, who used sound to restore balance in the energetic body and to prevent or heal illnesses. According to Pythagoras, health is harmony and illness is the imbalance of elements. He stated that to recover a healthy condition, it's necessary to reconcile all elements, and that reconciliation is possible through tuning. His understanding of musical wisdom explains the cathartic, enlightening, and healing power of tones. He created treatments based on harmonic frequencies, which harmonize the soul's feelings such as sorrow, rage, jealousy, fears, anxiety, excitement, depression, and violence.[2]

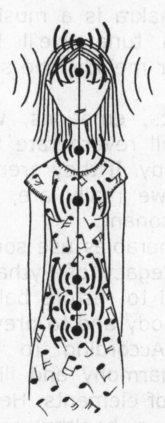

The body as a musical instrument.

Reestablishing the balance of the energetic bodies and having that reflected in the physical body may take a long time. That's why when there's an emergency or a disease already developed in the body, integrative oncology proposes to solve the problem at the physical level with an anticancer treatment and to engage other practices and therapies that need more time to restore health in the energetic bodies—to put the fire out while reinvigorating the whole system.

If the imbalance is long-term and has already settled in the body, it generally takes longer to restore balance. As in an economic crisis, if something has been brewing for a long time, we cannot expect a quick fix.

Yanina started to realize that having the tumor removed and then returning to her previous lifestyle didn't make sense. But it was difficult for her to see how to make healthy changes and get out of the rat race. I recommended a revitalization, tune-up, and self-knowledge program. Before she left my office, I thought it would be important for her to have an experience of feeling her body rather than just my explanations, so I invited her to do a conscious-breathing exercise.

"It's incredible, Laura, I feel so much more relaxed. Please teach me more."

During our next session, Yanina and I discussed the benefits of conscious breathing. I began by explaining that *breath* has the same root as *spirit*, which are both etymologically connected to the Sanskrit root *atma*, meaning essence, soul, or breath. In Hebrew, *ruah* means wind, blow, or spirit, and in Greek, *pneuma* has the same meaning. In their original meanings, both terms also signify the ability to listen to God. Sacred texts state that God created man out of dust and breathed into him the breath, or spirit, of life.

Our first breath takes place when we are born, and the last one when we die. That living breath, that vital force, is what keeps us alive and connected to the energy of the universe. With each breath, we exchange energy with the environment and bring the cosmos into circulation in the whole body.

The way we breathe when we're born is the best way to sustain that flow of energy. Watch babies breathe. With each breath, their lungs fill with air, push the diaphragm down, and inflate the abdomen. The bottom of their lungs is ventilated, and stagnant air is replaced by fresh air. Over time, we lose this natural ability to breathe and begin to use a smaller portion of our lung capacity.

The Sanskrit word *pranayama* refers to yogic breathing that concentrates and controls the *prana,* the life energy. There are many exercises that affect our body-mind.

Practice for Healthy Living

Take some quiet time for yourself.

Sit on a cushion on the floor or on a chair, with your spine upright. Place one hand on your chest and the other on your abdomen.

Close your eyes and breathe normally for a few seconds.

Then breathe in a little more deeply, as you count up to four, silently. Exhale slowly, as you count up to four.

While breathing in, inflate your abdomen, not your chest. It helps to relax your shoulders. If your shoulders are going up and down as you breathe, it means you're breathing with your chest rather than your abdomen.

You can also use your hands to tell you which part of your body and which muscles you're using to breathe. If you feel the hand on your abdomen extending out as you inhale, and not the hand on your chest, you are breathing deeply with your abdomen.

Breathe more slowly and deeply than normal. Lengthen the count of the exhalation to six, then to eight.

After doing this for some minutes, return to your normal breathing, counting four (in) and six (out), then four-four, and then breathe normally before opening your eyes.

Try this technique introducing a pause after each inhalation. Breath retention deepens relaxation even more as it stimulates the vagus nerve or cranial nerve X, which is a part of the nervous or parasympathetic system and induces relaxation.

When you begin these practices, it might feel uncomfortable or unnatural, but over time it will become easier.

This **deep or abdominal breathing** is used in yoga practices and allows the ventilation at the bottom of the lungs to get a better oxygenation affecting the whole body. More oxygen breathed in helps you feel less stress, less shortness of breath, and less anxiety.

Conscious breathing refers to any exercise we do while paying attention to our breathing. We can practice, for example, by silently reciting a mantra, or phrase, with every in- and out-breath (saying "in," "out"), or while counting each breath ("ten," "nine," and so on). Conscious breathing means focusing on the here and now, aligning body, mind, and spirit.

There are also deep breathing exercises developed in ancient India to quiet the mind and encourage awakening or enlightenment. Breathing this way helps manage stress, oxygenate tissues, and improve the body's alkalinity. Good breathing helps the alkalinization of blood by eliminating the excess of carbon dioxide, which acidifies it.

According to Indian philosophy, a central energy channel runs along the spine and is activated by deep breathing, moving vital energy up and down the spine. Practicing conscious breathing, we recharge with vital energy and integrate our body-mind so we feel the flowing unity within.

There is a close relation between breathing and emotions, and also between breathing and the body.

We can observe differences in our body when our breathing is labored and when it is calm. Calm breathing produces slow, wide movement of the chest, while anxious breathing produces short, rapid movements.

Breathing changes with our emotions, and at the same time,

emotions are changed through breathing. When we cry, for example, our breathing is labored. When we feel anxious, if we breathe deeply and slowly, we calm down. **Breathing helps us transform anxiety, stress, and feeling ill into ease, and helps calm the mind.** Breathing unites our subtle essence with matter; that is, mind is united with body.

Breathing is an alchemical process, allowing for the transmutation of gas molecules into solid molecules within our cells.

Just as in a campfire, when the fire, fed by oxygen, burns the wood and converts it into heat and ash, as oxygen arrives at the cellular level, a small "campfire" ignites in every cell of our body. The metabolic machinery within each cell, fed by the oxygen received through inhalation, transforms sugars into usable energy and carbon dioxide, which is then eliminated through the next exhalation.

When taking in oxygen, we oxygenate the mind, the body, and all their processes. When releasing carbon dioxide, we help the body alkalinize.

Breathing not only provides us with vital energy; it also helps release stagnant energy. Remember a stressful day when you didn't have time for even a short walk. Your body didn't have a chance to release the excess energy that accumulated, and you felt tired. At times like this, it's useful to practice **breathing exercises to discharge stagnant energy.**

After several breathing exercises, Yanina noticed changes in her body and mind. With her mind calmed, we were able to go more deeply into her journey of self-awareness. I explained that these exercises were going to help her feel better, tolerate the chemo, have less nausea and vomiting, and sleep better.

We began talking about the many characters that coexist inside each of us. Yanina was in identification with a dutiful workaholic, an insensitive, self-demanding tyrant. What about her sensitive side, the mother of her daughter and the compassionate caregiver for her dying mother?

Practice for Healthy Living

Sit comfortably in a quiet place where you're not likely to be interrupted, your back upright and your eyes gently shut. Put your cell phone on airplane mode.

Breathe in through your nostrils.

Exhale with your mouth open, as though you're misting a glass window. Or exclaim "Ahhhh!" as you breathe out.

Repeat this several times.

Before you open your eyes, scan your body from toe to head and observe how you feel.

It was important for Yanina to start training her mind, to learn through meditation to calm it down, be more spacious, and see more clearly. This would complement the work she'd begun a couple of weeks earlier with psychotherapy. I suggested that Yanina start with a basic meditation exercise.

Yanina returned a week later, and I asked how she was doing with her meditation experience. "Oh, Laura," she said. "I started working part-time and with such turmoil—the chemo, the work, and my daughter—I was only able to practice the first days! Then I just forgot about it. I noticed when I did it that it calmed me down, but when returned to the daily bustle, I lost track." I could feel that she was a little anxious and that putting meditation into practice was challenging for her. "I read about meditation in the newspapers. Would you say it's just fashionable or actually useful?" Her voice had a tone of frustration.

Practice for Healthy Living

Make yourself comfortable and ready to take some time to connect with yourself.

Sit in the same position you used while practicing mindful breathing.

With your eyes closed, observe your breathing. Then try to feel the sensations in your body. Then observe your mental activity.

With a consistent rhythm, repeat silently while inhaling, "I am," and while exhaling, "at peace."

If you get distracted by a thought and find your mind somewhere else, just become aware of it and invite your mind to return here and now by repeating, "I am at peace."

Start by practicing this **meditation** ten minutes a day. It's helpful to set an alarm clock to go off at the end of the time, so you can relax during the exercise and concentrate deeply. After some days, you can extend the meditation to fifteen or twenty minutes.[3]

I assured Yanina that meditation is not just fashionable, that these practices have been well established for thousands of years in Hinduism, Buddhism, and Christianity. All religions and spiritual traditions know the benefits of meditation and include some practices that lead the mind to a meditative state. Prayer, for example, not only opens new spiritual dimensions, it also leads the mind out of daily busyness into a quiet state. Other practices, such as rhythmical movement, can help us enter the mind of peace.

As religion began to lose its influence on everyday life, people stopped praying and connecting with their inner selves. Thanks to contact among cultures, other forms of meditation were introduced, and we now know that it isn't necessary to be a monk or a priest to meditate. With patience and dedication, anyone can meditate. Many people throughout the world practice meditation today.

There's no single way to meditate. Imagine an old-fashioned wagon with wooden wheels. Pay attention to one of the wheels and observe how the outer ring is joined to the center by spokes. There is movement in the periphery, yet the center is quiet. While we are busy rolling along in life, there is always a center where we can be at peace and reconnect with ourselves. It doesn't matter which spoke we choose to get there. What is important is to connect with the center, to quiet the mind, and to be open to whatever we experience.

Each of us can find a meditation appropriate for us, one we resonate with and enjoy practicing. Many forms of meditation require calmness and silence—controlled breathing, repeating a phrase or mantra, relaxing different parts of the body. But other forms involve movement, such as taiji or walking meditation.

Some Forms of Meditation

Mindfulness is a form of meditation focused on moment-by-moment awareness and living in a state of present-centered consciousness. Thoughts about the past—including judging and blaming oneself—or worries about the future can cause stress. While focusing on the present moment, you can calm yourself and restore balance in your immune system. You can practice while sitting, eating, walking, or any other activity. Mindfulness meditation has been used for thousands of years to reduce stress, anxiety, depression, and negative emotions.

In **focused meditation**, you put your full attention on an object, for example a flower or a candle flame. This anchors your attention and trains the mind to focus.

Through **visualization meditation**, specific images are conjured in the mind. Visualization may be guided by a person or by a recording to help us relax and create a meaningful image in our minds.

Transcendental meditation uses a mantra—a word or a phrase repeated in specific ways—to bring about focus, concentration, inner peace, and wellness.

Prayer is a form of meditation aimed at spiritual development. The meaning varies from religion to religion, as does the form of prayer. Some encourage connection with a particular spiritual being; others cultivate positive qualities such as wisdom and compassion.

Some traditions use **moving meditations,** which may be mindful walking, taiji, qigong, or yoga.

In recent decades, research studies have looked into the effects of meditation. Many are based on *mindfulness* meditation. These studies show that meditation promotes health and wellness. Generally speaking, people practice meditation to help calm and relax their body-mind.

Practice for Healthy Living

How can we practice **mindfulness?**

Place your full attention on what is happening now, without judging. You can focus on your breathing to anchor your mind in the present moment.

Judgments polarize our thinking—good or bad, right or wrong—creating an electromagnetic load in our brain, and our head *feels overloaded.* When we are free of judgments, the mind lightens and creates space for creative thinking.

While practicing mindfulness, when your mind gets distracted, simply observe how it fluctuates, how it gets distracted, or how it follows a thought, and bring it back to the present moment with kindness.

To practice mindfulness, you'll need:

• A quiet space and time with little or no distraction or disruption.

• A comfortable position, preferably not lying down, to help avoid falling asleep.

• Something to focus on. You can meditate with your eyes open or closed. If open, focus softly on a particular spot, for example a flower or another object, or the floor two to three feet in front of you. If your eyes are closed, focus on a feeling or an image.

• Observe without criticizing or judging. Try not to obsess over the content of thoughts. The mind generates thoughts all day long. It's used to doing so, and we usually encourage this by chitchat and other frivolous conversations, listening to the radio, watching TV, or sitting in front of our computer screen. Don't worry about whether you are doing it well (or not). As soon as you notice your mind becoming distracted, gently invite it to return to the object of your attention.

A daily meditation practice has many benefits:

- It reduces stress and helps manage uncertainty.
- It trains the mind to see more clearly, to have a wider perspective of what's happening to us, and helps us see the forest for the trees.
- It encourages inner peace, releasing thoughts and worries that might be tangled up in our heads.
- It helps us be more responsive to what's happening and avoid fixed reactions.
- It helps calm anxiety and improve the quality of sleep.
- It uplifts our mood and reduces depression.
- It reduces fatigue and chronic pain.
- It lowers blood pressure and symptoms of menopause.

In the case of Yanina and others suffering from cancer, there is evidence that meditation reduces the adverse effects of chemotherapy, particularly nausea and vomiting,[4] and stimulates the immune system.[5]

In the same way we learned to brush our teeth daily without conflict or debate, we can "brush our head" by practicing meditation daily, preventing the accumulation of "plaque" in the form of recurring thoughts and prevent illness caused by stress.

Meditation goes beyond relaxation and stress reduction. If we practice daily, we become more conscious of how we're living. **We meditate in order to connect with our inner wisdom, not to disconnect from the outside.** Through meditation we become more aware of the inner processes of the body and the experiences of our life. We develop an alert, fresh attitude, like a child discovering and marveling at life. We're no longer confined by habits and memories. We're bright, aware, and ready to act on what is before us. This is the way to a fuller, healthier, more present-centered life.

Do You Comb Your Thoughts Every Day?

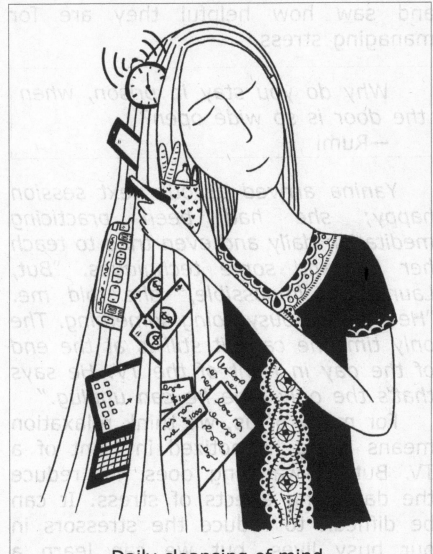

Daily cleansing of mind.

Clearing your mind daily helps free you from suffering.

Once I taught Yanina breathing and meditation practices, she practiced them and saw how helpful they are for managing stress.

> *Why do you stay in prison, when the door is so wide open?*
> —Rumi

Yanina arrived at our next session happy; she had been practicing meditation daily and even tried to teach her husband some techniques. "But, Laura, it's impossible," she told me. "He's always busy doing something. The only time he can sit still is at the end of the day in front of the TV. He says that's the only time he can unplug."

For many of us, we think relaxation means being hypnotized in front of a TV. But TV-watching does not reduce the damaging effects of stress. It can be difficult to reduce the stressors in our busy lives, but we can learn a **relaxation response** to balance them.

In chapter 3, "Why Do We Get Sick?" we saw that we have an "accelerator" and a "brake" system inside of us. The problems of everyday life, the demands of work, conflicts, traffic, air pollution, and feeling insecure, guilty, anxious, and afraid are all situations in which we "accelerate." If we don't slow down at least once a day to counter the effects of acceleration, our system will be unbalanced, and we'll feel hyperactive all the time. Our system stays on "alert," and the immune system and the PNIE network won't function properly. Eventually, the system will begin to fail.

The relaxation response is a condition of deep rest that balances stress. When you relax, your heartbeat slows, breathing deepens, blood pressure stabilizes, muscles soften, and the body starts to recover itself. Besides its soothing effect, relaxation increases focus and energy, helps us make better decisions, and encourages us to be more effective. When we come home from work stressed and take a moment to relax before preparing dinner, we're less likely to burn the food or have an accident in the kitchen. When we're sick, relaxation can help reduce pain.

By learning to relax, we slow down, counter everyday stress and other effects of acceleration, and return to balance, helping the PNIE network and immune system work properly. The relaxation response helps us cultivate resiliency, regain perspective, and rise again after falling down. Bamboo bends in the wind without breaking, then stands tall once again. Resiliency is not a trait some people have and others don't. It is an ability you can cultivate through relaxation exercises. With resiliency, we learn to cope with stress and keep ourselves healthy.[6] By practicing techniques like deep breathing, meditation, and yoga, we can calm ourselves every day.

There isn't a single relaxation technique that's best for everybody. The best technique for you is the one you resonate with, the one you're eager to practice, that fits in your schedule, helps you release everyday stress, and allows you to focus your mind. It can be useful to combine or alternate techniques, to keep your motivation fresh. One clue in choosing a relaxation technique is to become aware of how you respond to stress.

Do you respond to stress by **fighting?** Do you get angry or agitated or act violently—verbally or physically?

If this is the case, it would be better to choose a technique that calms you down, like meditation, deep breathing, guided visualization, or progressive muscle relaxation.

If, on the contrary, you activate the escape or flight mode when you feel stressed, if you get depressed, isolated, pensive, or hypnotized by your TV, practicing *any* activity to release stress and stimulate your nervous system can help. These include rhythmic exercises or movements, massage, mindful walking, or power yoga.

Practice for Healthy Living

Progressive muscle relaxation uses a two-step process in which you tense particular muscle groups and then release the tension.

Find a time and place to take a break. Breathe deeply and consciously a couple of times.

Pay attention to your right foot. Allow yourself to feel the sensations in that foot. Squeeze the muscles in your foot as tightly as you can. Count to ten while holding this tension, and then release it. Feel the tension ease. Continue feeling the release while breathing slowly.

When you feel ready, do the same with your left foot.

Move up through your body, tightening and relaxing part by part, following this sequence:

1. right foot, left foot
2. right calf, left calf
3. right thigh; left thigh
4. pelvis and gluteus
5. abdomen (suck it in)
6. chest
7. back
8. right arm, and then right forearm and hand
9. left arm, and then left forearm and hand
10. shoulders and neck
11. face (wrinkle your forehead and pucker your lips at the same time)

Practicing progressive muscle relaxation will also help you notice tension when it arises in daily life, and you can learn to relax body and mind to counterbalance the tension.

Practice for Healthy Living

Rhythmic exercises or movements refer to any physical activity that involves the arms and legs at the same time, such as running, walking, swimming, dancing, rowing, climbing, or practicing taiji. Releasing stress is most effective when practiced consciously. As with meditation, this means full awareness of the present moment.

While practicing these activities, focus attention on your feelings, arms, legs, and breathing, rather than your thoughts. If your mind gets distracted, gently bring it back and focus again on your breathing and what you feel.

If you're walking or running, focus on the soles of your feet, the sensations of each foot touching the ground, the air caressing your face, or the rhythm of your breathing.

If you've experienced trauma in the past, you might **freeze** when you face stress. Your body might be mostly motionless, although parts of it might move involuntarily, or you start to cough, feel shortness of breath, palpitations, or sweating. When you're in this situation, it's first necessary to activate your nervous system and *then* begin an appropriate relaxation technique. To activate your nervous system, choose a physical exercise or simply get up and walk. See if you want to continue this or change to another activity that might calm you down.

We all accumulate stress during daily life, regardless of which response to stress we express. Our neck, shoulders, and lower back normally accumulate stress, and there are exercises for moving these parts of the body that might be helpful to practice during the day to release stress.

Practice for Healthy Living

It's a good idea to do some practices to relax your neck and shoulders during the day. According to Tibetan Buddhism, the neck is the distributor of energy throughout our body. If the neck is blocked, energy doesn't flow between the head and the rest of the body.

Warning: If you have problems with your cervical vertebrae, such as arthritis, please consult your medical doctor before practicing the following exercise. And if your doctor allows you to practice, pay close attention not to squeeze the vertebrae while leaning your head backward.

Start with gentle and slow circular movements of your neck, for as long as you feel comfortable.

While you exhale, tuck your chin toward your chest, up to the point most easily reached.

As you inhale, lift your head up and tilt it backward, so the chin is pointing toward the sky without overstretching or hurting yourself. (If you have *any* problems with your cervical vertebrae, only hold your head upright; do not lean it back.)

Inhale and hold your breath for a moment; then exhale as you move your chin back toward your chest.

Return your head to the center.

Now, as you inhale, tilt your head to the right, as though you want to lay it on a cushion on your right shoulder. Breathe in, in that position, observing what you can loosen to let the head get a little closer to the right shoulder.

Very slowly, as you exhale again, return your head to the center.

Repeat this movement, this time to the left.

After practicing this movement down, up, left, and right, rotate your head again, and notice if there are any changes from when you did this at the beginning of the exercise.

Return your head to the center. Stay still for a few moments, breathing comfortably and allowing yourself to notice any new sensations arising in your body.

When you feel ready, return to your activities.

The best way to maintain an anti-stress, relaxing practice is to incorporate it into your daily routine. It can be difficult to find free time during the day, so it's easiest if you practice while also doing something else. For example, once you've learned to practice conscious breathing, you can do it while you're on the bus or the train. Once you've learned rhythmic exercising, you can practice as you clean house, mow the lawn, walk to an appointment, walk the dog, or walk up the stairs. You can practice mindful awareness while washing the dishes, paying full attention to the water temperature and the textures of the glasses, plates, and utensils.

Scheduling practice times once or twice a day can also be useful. When you wake up in the morning is a good time, before you're overtaken by responsibilities. You'll feel happy for the accomplishment and for starting the day connecting with yourself.

Learning relaxation techniques and incorporating them into your life takes time. To help make it easier in the beginning, schedule some passive relaxation therapy, such as acupuncture or reflexology, once a week.

Yanina was enthusiastic. In just a few weeks, she was practicing every day, alternating between meditation and breathing exercises, and doing this was helping her better endure the chemo. She observed that others receiving chemotherapy were suffering more. She also felt calmer, but she did find herself thinking and worrying from time to time, and couldn't get certain thoughts out of her head. "They're more powerful than I am," she confided.

Still, Yanina was no longer prey to her thoughts and was becoming aware of how the mind functions. One of the fruits of her meditation was the ability to see more clearly, to observe her thoughts.

If we pay attention to the flow of our thoughts, we can notice when our mind is active, dealing with a train of thoughts, and when it's quiet and calm. We can also observe when we're brooding over something that won't leave us alone. We learn to distinguish between positive thoughts, which give us feelings and sensations of well-being, and negative thoughts, which lead us toward suffering.

Meditation practice helps us become aware of our mind's activities and contents and how to calm the mind and choose healthy thoughts.

More than 90 percent of our thoughts are not new. We repeat the same thoughts over and over. **Positive thoughts give rise to healthy attitudes;** negative thoughts have the opposite effect. If we reinforce negative circuits, over time they'll instill in us unhealthy habits, and eventually we'll get sick.

Gandhi reminded us:

Carefully watch your thoughts,
for they become your words.

Manage and watch your words,
for they will become your actions.

Consider and judge your actions,
for they have become your habits.

Acknowledge and watch your
habits,
for they shall become your values.

Understand and embrace your
values,
for they become your destiny.[7]

Words—spoken words and written words—have their own power. That's why it's important to nourish ourselves with healthy words.

One way to do this is to cultivate kind thoughts. If our mind were a garden, you wouldn't throw trash there. To keep the mind fertile, it's necessary to track what comes in—news, media, gossip, judgments—and allow space for inspiration and creativity.

Transforming negative thoughts by focusing on them is next to impossible. **The only way to change negative events or situations is by reinforcing positive ones.** We need to choose thoughts that calm us and help us stay in the present moment. We can tend our mind's garden with daily readings from sacred texts, inspiring writings, and poems. These words will displace our negative thoughts.

In addition to becoming aware of negative content we receive from outside sources, it's important to observe conversations we have with ourselves. If we repeat "I can't," "I'm useless," "I'm wrong," or "I don't know how," we'll never go forward. Try to change negative patterns into healthier ones.

Healthy phrases include those that empower us and give us hope. Instead of "I can't," try saying, "I know it's difficult, yet I'll try." Speak in a way that encourages you. The mind doesn't understand negative instructions, like "I do not want to smoke." The mind hears, "I want to smoke." A healthy rephrasing might be, "I want to take care of my body."

Using Healthy Phrases in Everyday Life

When dealing with addictions to tobacco or food, it's useful to accompany a healthy, encouraging phrase with a positive action.

For example, when you crave a cigarette, try instead to practice ten conscious breaths. Instead of repeating, "I don't want to smoke," say, "I'm breathing in fresh air." If the addiction is to food, practice ten conscious breaths, and instead of saying, "I don't want to eat more sweets," say, "I want to follow a healthy diet."

Choose your words carefully whether you're speaking to yourself (internal dialogue) or with others. There are people we habitually speak negatively to, criticizing others, noting how bad things are in the world. Negative images arise, which express in our bodies as stress molecules. It's important to spend less time with certain people or in certain places. When necessary, change the topic.

Sometimes when we don't expect it, we receive negative news. This happens in the health sector, where the effect of words can be especially impactful. Some in our profession don't choose "the most perfect or positive words." They impart information with little concern for its effect, as when a doctor says, "Your cancer will return," and some months later the person develops a metastasis. Or the doctor who says, "You'll only live six months," and the person dies six months later. Did the doctor foresee the future, or did the person believe the doctor's words so literally that the body obeyed? How can we explain that, under similar circumstances, another person doesn't relapse and lives many more years?

> *Be impeccable with your word.*
> —Don Miguel Ruiz, *The Four Agreements*[8]

What can we do when we unexpectedly receive one of these harmful messages? The best we can do is to center ourselves and try to avoid being affected. For example, when you're going to a doctor's appointment, imagine that you're the CEO of a company en route to a meeting with your attorneys. Each lawyer has a specialty but lacks the big picture. In the same way, your doctor is a specialist in disease and its treatment but doesn't know about some of the other conditions contributing to your illness—emotional, familial, or spiritual conflicts. It's important to take into account each specialist's advice and consider that point of view along with that of other specialists. To support your global vision, it's useful to have the support of a doctor devoted to you as a whole—body, mind, and spirit.

Yanina appreciated this explanation. She remembered many examples in her life that confirmed the power of words. She left my office eager to read *The Four Agreements.*

Practice for Healthy Living

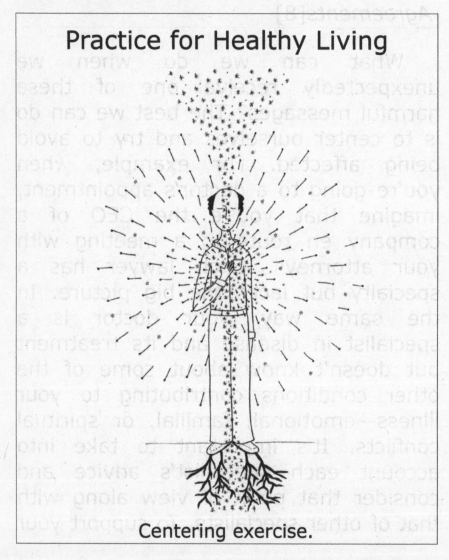

Centering exercise.

Standing or sitting, take a couple of deep breaths and then focus on your feet. Imagine your feet are the roots of a tree growing slowly, downward into the soil.

Now imagine a beam of nourishing light coming up from the center of the earth, entering your feet, and continuing up to your heart. At the same time, imagine a beam of light coming down from the sky, entering through the crown of your head and continuing down to your heart, where it joins with the beam of light coming up from the earth.[9]

Put one hand on your chest, and with each breath, be aware of the energy radiating from your chest and filling your whole body. Now imagine that energy expanding to fill the room, then the building, the neighborhood, the city, the country, the planet, and the universe.

Centered within your expanded energy, you're ready to have an encounter with another person. Allow only their nourishing energy to enter your sphere.

This centering exercise helps you prepare for an appointment with a doctor, a lawyer, a meeting with your boss, or even with your partner, especially when you need to discuss a difficult topic.

Yanina arrived at our next session with mixed feelings. She was happy her chemo was going well and the tumor was now small enough to go ahead with surgery. But her operation was coming up in two weeks, and she was afraid "of everything—the anesthesia, the surgery, how my breasts will look. I don't know if I'm strong enough!"

I said her fear of surgery and of all the unknowns is common and even sensible. I insisted on the importance of being as prepared as possible in body, mind, and spirit to be calm for the surgery, as this would help her get better results. I used an image I love—Jesus walking on the water—to show that miracles take place when conditions are favorable, in this case that wind and water were calm. When our thoughts (wind) and emotions (water) are calm, the impossible becomes possible.

I encouraged Yanina to calm her mind with meditation before the surgery and to work with her emotions to be prepared for the challenge. There's a close relationship between emotions and bodily functions. We can no longer say emotions are in the head or even that they're born in the brain. Emotions have a significant somatic component that combines muscular and visceral components that can't be separated from mental reactions.

Each emotion affects a specific region of the body, and this is true in all cultures and at all ages. Pain and anxiety usually affect the heart of those suffering from loss. Research shows an increase of heart attacks—even fatal ones—following the death of a loved one. We say, "She died of sadness." Anger activates our head; depression takes away the strength of our arms and legs. Feelings in the throat and digestive system are related to anxiety. Fear, anxiety, and shame are often felt in the belly. "I have a knot (or a brick) in my stomach." "It's indigestible."

The body has a much more developed intelligence than we'd thought, and it conditions much of our conduct. In recent years, the connection between conduct, mood, and gut health has been clearly shown, and **the gut is now considered a second brain.**

Functions performed by the brain include memory, moods, and intelligence. In fact, *our nervous and immune systems also have memory.* Two-thirds of our immune system is located in the abdomen, surrounding the digestive system.[10] Regarding moods, most of the serotonin, the antidepressant molecule linked with happiness, is produced in the abdomen, not in the brain.[11] How many times do we make decisions based on gut feelings?

Understanding the abdomen as a second brain and bearing in mind that it's the reservoir of many emotions, we see the importance of eating a healthy diet and maintaining a healthy digestive tract by moving our bowels regularly.

The way we deal with emotions is significant.

Yanina's interest perked up. She remembered that as a child, she'd suffered stomachaches whenever she got nervous. And the last few days, she was having digestive issues, feeling bloated after eating and suffering from diarrhea, which she thought must have been due to something she ate. While telling me this, she realized it had started when she'd learned the date of her surgery. "What can I do with my fear and emotions?"

I offered an overview of how to deal with emotions and some tips to prepare for surgery. To maintain balance within, we need a healthy **coordination between our two brains, what we think and what we feel.** Self-knowledge techniques help us to take into account the way we think and the way we deal with emotions and to develop emotional intelligence (EI).[12]

Researchers have come to recognize that emotional intelligence is as important as intellectual intelligence (intelligence quotient, IQ)—perhaps more important. People with high IQs but scant relationship skills due to emotional outbursts have difficulty achieving objectives. Without emotional intelligence, feelings dominate our lives. Do you ever feel that anger or depression push you around? Do you ever respond impulsively, saying something you wish you hadn't? Do you feel sleepy, without feeling, without getting angry or feeling deeply happy? Has anyone ever told you you're like a machine or a robot? Do you feel life is an emotional roller coaster? All these situations indicate poorly developed emotional intelligence.

Thanks to neuro- and PNIE-plasticity, all human qualities can be modified. Our personality is associated with specific neural circuits that we've learned and repeat because (at least at one time) they've worked for us. Negative emotions, such as anger, annoyance, and hostility, are habits we can change to positively influence outcomes. In general, anger and annoyance are the external expression of something deeper—sometimes fear. **The gateway to happiness is to cultivate a more trustful heart.**

Practice for Healthy Living

Whenever you feel annoyed, ask yourself:

"What am I afraid of?"

"What do I need that I'm not getting?"

You can also ask these questions of someone else: "What do you need?" "How can I help you?" These questions can help the exchange be more nourishing for both of you.

Emotional intelligence, or EI, has nothing to do with intellectual capacity, but with self-esteem, self-awareness, empathy, and compassion, all of which play important roles in the way we live. When we develop emotional intelligence, we learn:

- to be more conscious of ourselves, our thoughts, feelings, and emotions
- to know our strengths and weaknesses
- to identify, express, and deal with our feelings by developing empathy
- to become aware of impulses, to recognize frustration, and to delay gratification

- to cope better with anxiety and stress[13]

By cultivating emotional intelligence, we come to understand, manage, and express our emotions in healthy, constructive ways. EI also helps us recognize and respond to the others' emotions appropriately. We learn to develop attentive listening and ask questions using appropriate words in a constructive tone.

People with good emotional development are able to communicate clearly and maintain good relationships in their work and family. They also recover from difficult situations, encourage themselves, find solutions to problems, and achieve what is important to them.

Emotions have been identified as "messengers of the soul."[14] An emotion appears to bring information, and it's important to listen to it. In the body, emotions speak by means of a molecular cascade. When we allow an emotion to express itself, we're allowing the flow of millions of information molecules. The body keeps healthy when this information is transmitted fluently and fluidly.[15] The healthy expression of our emotions helps us align and integrate body, mind, and spirit.

How can we cope with negative emotions? First of all, we can be present with the impulse without either acting it out or suppressing it. Letting an emotion take us over can create a shock that has the magnitude of an earthquake, impacting our body and spirit adversely. If we are angry and don't register it in our consciousness, that's also problematic. And if we suppress it and instead wear a smile on our face, the "anger molecules" stay inside us and are harmful.

Just as we avoid insulting others, we should avoid using destructive language against ourselves.

If this happens over and over, we build a large dam inside ourselves, and it takes a lot of energy to keep our emotions suppressed. Repeated suppression of emotions produces chronic stress in the body. And as we saw in chapter 3, "Why Do We Get Sick?" it makes us more vulnerable to disease.[16] Thoughts and emotions might play a primary role in the development of chronic illness. Even when we follow a healthy lifestyle—eating a nutritious diet, exercising regularly, and sleeping well—emotions exert a great power on our body.

Suppressed emotions accumulate in the body as information molecules, and cells store in memory how many times certain circuitries have been triggered.[17] In other words, the way we responded emotionally in the past will influence the way we'll respond today. Neural pathways already grooved will be favored, and we're likely to have the same reaction time after time. Favoring certain circuits also determines some of our body's postures and habits, for example, whether we stand with our head held high or bent forward. Just as the proper functioning of a car depends on the flow of fuel, without spurting or stagnation, our emotional expression depends on the flow of information molecules.

We cannot separate health from emotions. The fact that uncontrolled expressions of emotion or the accumulation of suppressed negative emotions adversely affect health suggests that emotional freedom can help us recover good health. It's important to factor our emotional state in our health plan.[18]

How can we get our emotions to flow in a healthy way? There are techniques that can help us live more calmly and cope more effectively with whatever arises.

Practicing meditation, we learn to be more present, clear our mind, and become more adept at coping with negative emotions. We become mindful of what's happening in the present moment, without judgment—which in fact is the basis for emotional intelligence. Being present helps us detect emotions, judgments, and intuitions and cultivate positive feelings, which take their own place, ousting negative emotions. Meditation encourages the arising of compassion and the natural goodness we each have inside us. **Compassion is not just**

sentimentality or holding someone's hand. It's a good medicine.[19]

Practice for Healthy Living

The traffic light technique helps impulses flow through us without causing damage. When you feel angry or anxious, how can you coordinate your thoughts with your feeling? It can be useful to think of a traffic light.

1. **Red light.** Stop, calm down, and think before acting.

2. **Amber light.** Talk about the problem, giving words to how you feel. Propose a positive goal. Think about several possible outcomes and their consequences.

3. **Green light.** Move forward and put the best plan into action!

When we have a negative emotion, it can be difficult to process it as it arises. But if we're trained and can recognize the seed of a negative emotion the moment it surfaces, we can channel its energy and help it flow through us promptly, without leaking. Other techniques for working with emotions include "Traffic Light" and "Letting Go."

With practice, you'll be able to identify negative emotions as they arise and accompany rather than resist or deny them. After the dust settles, you'll be able to process them so that nothing remains stuck inside. **It's important to try to understand the message your emotions bring before "letting go" of them.** Find a quiet place and "listening" to your body, *feel* any sensations associated with this emotion. You can also explore thoughts, images, and memories that arise. This isn't always easy. Take whatever time is needed to try to get a feeling for what "message" is being conveyed to you from within.

As was said in the science-fiction movie *Interstellar,* referring to Newton's third law,[20] "To move forward, we have to leave something behind."[21] If we want to move forward in life, the clue is to let loose old resentments, thought patterns that lead us around dizzying mental labyrinths, possessive and controlling relationships that don't allow us to be....

Practice for Healthy Living

What would it be like to walk without the backpack filled with heavy stones we carry every day?

Let go of resentments, anger, and frustration to lighten the load. Find ways to express these feelings through your body, as though you were giving away old clothes or throwing a stone into the middle of a lake. As you do this, say loudly, "I let _____ go!" Do you feel lighter?

Forgiveness is another tool for letting go. It releases you from far more than the individual with whom you have a painful history. According to Carolyn Myss, "Forgiveness releases you from an ego state of consciousness that clings to a need for justice built around the fear of being humiliated, based on prior experiences of humiliation."[22]

Gratitude is another powerful tool. When we give thanks, we acknowledge the positive side of what we have, what we are, and what's happening to us. When we give thanks, the body relaxes and produces wellness-enhancing substances. Like compassion and forgiveness, **gratitude is good medicine.**

> Everything is a gift. The degree to which we are awake to this truth is a measure of our gratefulness, and gratefulness is a measure of our aliveness.
> —Brother David Steindl-Rast, *Jesus and Lao Tzu: The Parallel Sayings*

What happens when a negative emotion arises while we're in the midst of a conflict? While coping with a tense situation, how shall we manage our impulses? The point is not to suppress conflict, but to act in advance to resolve misunderstandings or differing points of view before they get out of control. **Nonviolent communication (NVC)** is a useful technique. It teaches how to name *feelings, needs, and requests,* based on listening attentively to others, giving each person the time and space needed to express themselves without blaming, judging, or putting them down.[23]

Nonviolent Communication (NVC)[24]

What I want in my life is compassion,
a flow between myself and others
based on a mutual giving from the heart
—Marshall B. Rosenberg

When we're in a conflict, NVC can help us express our needs and listen to others, instead of just reacting.

NVC invites us to give attention to our needs and the needs of others and to be aware of situations that affect us adversely. Being present allows us to know what we think and feel and to identify and express what we expect from a situation. Since NVC focuses on attentive listening, not only to others but also ourselves, it encourages respect, empathy, and the opening of our hearts and helps prevent conflicting needs from escalating into violence.

NVC's three basic steps are simple but transformative:

1. **Observe** and detect the problem, the thing that's affecting you, and **articulate** this observation.
2. Express **how I feel** in relation to this situation without judgment or blame.
3. Say **what I need** in order to avoid discomfort from that situation.

As Yanina listened to my words, she remembered a recent argument she'd had with her husband. He was an hour late picking her up from a pediatrician's appointment, and she took advantage of the situation by reproaching him about many of the things she was angry about. The tenor of the exchange escalated, and they ended up not talking to each other.

We recalled that situation and used role-playing to help her see how she might use NVC the next time. Yanina played herself, bombarding him from the outset: "Why are you late? Don't you see...! You always do the same thing!" Her accusatory tone triggered her husband's defensiveness, and the fight escalated.

Using NVC, the conversation might have gone like this: "Juan, when our agreement for you to pick me up at 3:00 was not fulfilled [observation and the articulation of actual facts], I began to feel anxious and upset [using words descriptively, without judgment or blame]. It's important to me that we fulfill our agreements, and when something unexpected arises, that we call each other [express needs]."

Expressing what we *feel* (rather than what we think) prevents the listener from responding critically; you can't really question what someone feels. The listener could refute the other's *thoughts* and even say something accusatory back. Engaging empathy helps us open our hearts and speak from a place of love and respect.

In recent years, new techniques for dealing with emotions have appeared. It is becoming more common for mind-body therapies to recognize emotions as an integral part of the health-disease process. Many of these techniques are based on the wisdom of ancient cultures, and include singing, dancing, and exercise—using movement and massage to release suppressed emotions. When this happens, people experience a "great liberation," and newly available energy arises.

Emotional Freedom Techniques (EFT), also known as *tapping,* is like "psychological acupuncture" and can be used to get free of negative emotions.[25] EFT uses acupuncture points, but instead of needles, the person simply taps on the points repeatedly. While stimulating these points, the person thinks about a certain problem—a traumatic event, strong emotion, addiction, pain, or anxiety, and repeats this healthy and empowering reminder: "Even though I'm angry, I deeply and completely love and accept myself." This helps remove short-circuits or emotional blocks and restores internal balance.[26]

Yanina liked the practice of tapping and began using it to free herself from fear as her surgery date was nearing. For the next two weeks, she also took time every day for meditation, exercise, and massage, and she arrived for her surgery much calmer. The operation was a success, and she was discharged promptly. Pathology tests showed that the tumor had responded well. For her, the worst of the anticancer treatment was over.

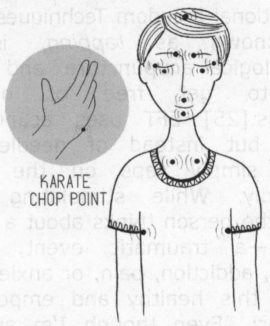

KARATE
CHOP POINT

Emotional freedom techniques (EFT).

Months later, Yanina came to see me expressing a new concern: "I'm feeling well now, Laura, and I don't know how to make this any clearer to my friends, family, and colleagues. I suffered a tsunami, but now, according to doctors, the possibility of a cure is high, and I'm focusing on my life and not on my disease. People keep looking at me as if I'm about to die at any moment."

Yanina had come a long way. I was touched when I remembered the day we met, when she just wanted the tumor removed so she'd be able to return to work. She had done—and she was doing—remarkably well recovering her health. She had learned to connect with her body, take on healthy habits, calm her mind, conquer her fears, align herself energetically, develop ways to bond with others while staying respectful to herself, and become more affectionate and compassionate, and this healthful approach to life had led her to devote more time to self-care. Energy poured from her toward her small daughter and her husband, and she gave priority to her family's well-being, creating quality moments and setting healthy limits to her work.

The image and sense of *cancer* that had overwhelmed her when she received the diagnosis were more about the things people say about cancer, its social stigma, rather than the disease discovered in her body. There's still a lot of ignorance about the variety of diseases represented by the word *cancer.* Many people conjure the image of someone suffering from cancer as though it is a single disease—always terminal—even those with an excellent cure rate diagnosed in time.

Now Yanina could see the monster that had frightened her as a friend that had accompanied her along this path to self-knowledge. It can be difficult to express this feeling to others, who know little about the disease or how changes in lifestyle can affect the health-disease axis. This disease, even when cured, often leaves a stigma that can make even those who no longer have a tumor suffer from the label—*cancer.* **Collective ignorance and beliefs can make us suffer, even when we're no longer ill.**

I advised Yanina to distinguish between those who were with her for her healthy change and believe in her transformation and those who remain skeptical. It's important to be surrounded by people who believe in you and your commitment to healthy life habits. This, I said, would help her maintain and build on all that she's learned. Yanina continued to flourish[27] and became an exemplar of a conscious, healthy lifestyle for many of the people around her.

When I saw Yanina again the following year, she seemed a different person. She had finally changed jobs. Over time, she became aware that she felt really good while helping other people, and she received a job offer where she could do that. "I'm happy; I feel more alive. Doing something I really like makes me so happy."

Connecting with something that gives meaning to our lives is essential to feeling vital and keeping healthy. We often find ourselves living a life that's more about what the society expects of us than what's important or makes sense to us. How many people suddenly realize that although they're successful from a professional and social point of view, they feel empty inside?

Practice for Healthy Living
What is your purpose?

What gives meaning to your life? Are you connected with that?

While you journey along the path toward self-knowledge, it can be useful to keep a journal. Write down those things you discover, the things that surprise you—perhaps a dream or a coincidence that might appear.

As with connect-the-dot children's books, these writings may point the way forward and help you see where you're going, to reconnect with the things that give your life meaning.

The key is to notice what makes you enthusiastic, fully alive. Stay connected with your *feelings,* and recognize when your body bustles with pleasure molecules. When a person buys new clothes, it's often to satisfy the ego. What I'm describing is more like the feeling you have after playing with your child or grandchild, gathering flowers you'd planted, dancing to your favorite song, writing a story, or painting a mandala. When we connect with the sense of aliveness, our Self experiences the fullness of life, and our body feels like a wave of expansion, enthusiasm, and complete happiness.

***Feeling* gives us the clues to stay on our path.** To be aligned, to keep the energy flowing inside ourselves and have our bodies shimmer, we need to be in our emotional axis and **unify our thinking, feeling, and acting.** The mind, the emotions, and the body are like horses pulling a carriage. To get them to ride in tandem, they all need to pull in the same direction. Thus, the driver—our soul, our wisest part—can move forward and continue toward what it came into this life to discover.

Enthusiasm: Having a God Inside Us

Enthusiasm is the movement of the soul by something that delights us, something we truly admire.

For ancient Greeks, *enthusiasm* meant "the god within."

An enthusiastic person is someone guided by wisdom and the force of a god, capable of making the impossible possible.

If we think and say what we feel, if we do what we feel and think, the carriage will move forward without obstacles. But how often do we say something or do something to please others, to avoid being frowned upon, to be included?

If the mind pulls toward one side, the emotions toward another, and the body in yet a different direction, the carriage cannot go forward and is in danger of overturning. The soul might pull on the reins to help us realign and regain the way of coherence. The soul redirects us through messages, for example when we want to do something or go in a certain direction and nothing comes of it, that might be to tell us, "That is not the way."

How many times do we insist on taking a certain path or making a certain choice that the soul knows will lead to suffering? The ego has the reins and insists on driving.

With conscious body practices like yoga, Eutony, or Sensory Awareness, we can *experience* **body-mind unity.** We observe our body's responses and become aware of feelings and sensations. This sense of integration stimulates our creativity and encourages us to express our potential. From a biological view, these practices reflect the activity of the autonomic nervous system, and both the conscious and nonconscious parts of the body are revealed as they affect and guide our movements, postures, breathing, and mental and emotional states.

Say What You Do and Do What You Say

How many times do we feel we don't want something, but accept doing it anyway?

How often do we think one thing and then act the opposite?

It's critical that body-mind work together as an inseparable team.

Let thinking, feeling, and acting cohere within yourself!

Our mind-body-spirit is full of intelligence, the same intelligence that allowed us to create a highly complex body from the union of our mother's ovule and our father's sperm, the same intelligence that allows us to know the moment—when everything is dark and we seem to be in a blind alley—to pass through the birth canal, the same intelligence keeps us healthy for so many years, dealing with stress, bacteria, viruses, fungi, radiation, pollution, and emotional tsunamis.

The mind-body knows what to do, and it's important to reactivate that intelligence, to make it more conscious every day. Breathing helps us conjoin body and mind; meditation helps us calm the mind; emotional cleansing techniques help us keep our energy flowing; and prayer and contemplative reflection help us align with our highest purpose. Integrating what we think with what we feel and do allows our soul to express itself.

The flow of our body-mind-spirit is like water, constantly changing, with limitless forms of expression. We are made of the same raw material as a forest, a mountain, or a stream. Our body is already a part of nature and can tune into our innate intelligence and awaken its own fullness. Connecting with nature calms us down and offers deep satisfaction.

Aligning with Our Purpose Is a Form of Prayer

There are many ancient forms of prayer. One that is seldom practiced nowadays is based on feeling. This kind of prayer uses our natural ability to communicate directly with universal intelligence, to attract what we want and take an active part in the process. It is based on "recognizing God within" and allows us to feel empowered. It's distinguished from other forms of prayer, which are based on seeking assistance from an external higher being.

Gregg Braden, scientist and author of many best sellers, encourages this form of prayer—which involves all our senses as a full body, mind, and spirit experience.

Silently, place your hands somewhere comfortable, perhaps on your chest or in another place on your body that feels expansive, as though seeking connection with the invisible.

Feel your body as though your prayer has already been heard. Feel in your body for a sense of satisfaction, joy, peace, and completeness. According to the law of resonance, you are taking an active part in the achievement of your purpose, attracting everything and everyone you need to fulfill your goal. Practicing this form of prayer keeps you actively engaged in your healing.[28]

Practice for Healthy Living

Walk barefoot on the grass.
This can help you feel more balanced. You are literally "earthing." Walking on the earth, you replenish your body with the earth's electrons.[29]

Yanina was able to see how the disease had shown her the imbalance in her life and was a call to recover her health. The organ that showed the illness, her breast, was evidence of a great misalignment of body, mind, and spirit. Now she felt more integrated and balanced with everything around her, her family, and work. She liked extending this feeling to include nature. Yanina was now clear that *tuning up* had brought her a long way to recovering her health, and it would continue to be the way to stay healthy.

Take-Home Message

Collective ignorance makes us suffer because people keep believing we are ill and act accordingly.

Health and emotions are closely related. Positive thoughts give rise to opportunities for health and growth.

We need good coordination between the thinking and feeling brains.

Emotional intelligence helps us understand, manage, and express our emotions in a healthy, constructive way.

Connecting with something that gives meaning to our lives is essential to feel alive and stay healthy.

It's essential to introduce new practices into our everyday life to cleanse our thoughts and emotions.

Conscious breathing is helpful to ease anxiety and calm the mind.

We practice meditation to reconnect with our inner wisdom, not to disconnect from the world.

Chapter 10

CAN CANCER BE A WAKE-UP CALL?

If we listen carefully, we can hear a voice trying to get our attention and wake us up....

It takes courage to answer the call, and if you choose to do so, your hero's journey begins.

—SPRING WASHAM

Fabiana, a renowned gastroenterologist and chief of service in a hospital, came to see me after breast cancer surgery. She was very concerned with the diagnosis, and although she was recovering quickly after surgery, she decided to take a leave for a few weeks. She told me, "I know this is trying to tell me something, but I feel lost. The only thing that comes to mind is, 'Stop the world, I want to get off.'"

Reading the pathology report, I emphasized to her that the cancer was *in situ,* i.e., it was incipient, not invasive, and there was no risk of it spreading to other parts of her body. I calmed her down by explaining that considering the stage in which her cancer was discovered and following its removal, it may well have been cured. I agreed, however, that it was good to take her alarm signal seriously.

During our first appointment, she began to recognize that she'd been placing her body under a lot of stress and wasn't all that happy. She felt guilty she'd let herself get carried away by all the work stress, leaving little time for herself or her family. She knew she couldn't continue like that, but felt confused.

I told her she was in the initial stages of a process of awakening. **Cancer can be a wake-up call,** a call to go beyond what's familiar and known, **to enter a path of self-knowledge.** I suggested that during the week she think about what she finds pleasant and what stresses her, and write it down in a notebook.

Fabiana took the first steps, and she came to our second session with a clearer mind, but still with mixed feelings. On the one hand, she felt compelled to return to her habitual rhythm. I told her that was her ego acting like a despot, demanding she continue as CEO. On the other hand, she recognized that that lifestyle was enslaving her. *"I had to write down how little leisure time I have, how little time I spent with my teenage son in the past months, and how much I'm not at home."* The voice from the depth of her soul was beginning to be heard, asking her to see that she was more than a successful physician. She *was practicing* her profession, but as a person *she was* much more. She was also a woman, a wife, a mother, a friend, a daughter, and a sister.

Her process was accelerated by her health crisis. Crises, whether at a personal, family, social, or global level, can be seen as a danger or as an opportunity to wake up and to rethink our life. Philosophers have been raising this question for centuries.

The attitude we take about a crisis will determine how we deal with it.

Most important is to face it with energy, hope, and optimism.

Faced with a crisis, someone not ready for change sees everything as adversity. Faced with a cancer diagnosis, for example, some people feel it's a dead end. For them, crisis equals danger. In contrast, those open to change, who understand that we are intelligent and adaptable beings, will face what's happening from a different perspective and see cancer as an opportunity to change, to transform themselves and their world.

Crisis: Danger or Opportunity?

A crisis is an emergency and entails making critical decisions. It shows that a system isn't working properly and needs to change. Crises arise unexpectedly and cause uncertainty.

Most people associate crises with chaos, misfortune, and danger. A crisis can, however, make us aware of what's not working and offer the opportunity to transform it.

The first step, a big one, is to dare to answer the call and be open to change.

> *I can't change the direction of the wind, but I can adjust my sails to always reach my destination.*
> —Jimmy Dean

Wake-up calls in life have a variety of ringtones, and we often don't hear them until they hurt. Cancer can bring intense physical as well as emotional pain. For Fabiana, it was difficult to accept vulnerability now that she was standing on the opposite side—as patient and not as doctor.

Pain is a part of life, although the reason for it is still a mystery. Believing that if we live in a healthy way we're going to live without pain is illusory. Some people say it's like thirst or hunger, a body's warning device telling us how we are. **Pain makes us pay attention to the situation we're in and gives us the possibility of becoming more conscious.**

What For?

> *Suffering happens, it is part of life. When I accept suffering as part of the mystery of life, I stop asking myself "why me?" and start asking "what for?"*
> —Father Anselm Grün

Times of pain offer us the potential to radically transform. To do this, we must go *through* the pain, deep into its roots to discover its cause. If we expect to relieve pain without feeling it or looking into its root causes, it will probably come back later, with the same appearance or in a different form. **The only way out is through,** to face what is happening consciously, to understand the message being offered.

There's a difference between pain and suffering. Pain is inevitable, but how much we suffer depends on our attitude. If we go through pain consciously, without complaining or feeling like a victim, and if we "get the message," we'll be stronger afterward. If we worship our pain or make it the enemy, the oppressor, we won't learn anything, and we'll probably suffer even more.

Fabiana wanted to know more. She told me, "I understand what you're saying, that crisis can be an opportunity, that pain can bring more or less suffering depending on one's attitude, but help me understand 'waking up.' Waking up to what?"

Practice for Healthy Living

Imagine you're in a telephone booth, the kind that used to be everywhere, with a door that closes. While you're in the phone booth, someone puts a red balloon in. No matter where you stand, you keep seeing it. It's always in view.

Now imagine the phone booth magically getting bigger and bigger until it reaches the size of an airplane hangar. The red balloon is still there, but there's so much more space. You can move freely, barely noticing the balloon.

The same can be true of pain. We can be stuck to our pain and let it fill our whole life till we suffer permanently. Or we can expand the space we reside in, allowing other thoughts, emotions, and experiences to enter, and even though we still have to live with our pain, the suffering will be much less.

I shared my view that in spite of the physical and emotional pain, **a cancer diagnosis can be a wake-up call.** We can choose to ignore it and keep sleeping, or listen to it and commit ourselves to waking up and facing what life is offering. **Cancer is an invitation to awaken, to set forth on a road of self-knowledge.** Knowing ourselves, we can live more fully each day.

This wake-up call is a warning, inviting us to take off our mask and realize who we really are. Most of us identify more with what we do than who we are. As we saw in chapter 8, "Do I Know Who I Am?," our ego identifies with one of our many inner characters and thinks one is the principal actor. We see ourselves as the CEO, accountant, architect, mother, or son.

When the ego's identification is far from who we really are, our soul implores us to wake up to the rest of ourselves. To be complete beings, we need to integrate ego and soul. **Waking up is a call to enter a spiritual journey, a meeting with our soul.**

"That's exactly what's happening to me," Fabiana said. *"I've always seen myself as the leader, and now that I'm on leave, I feel lost. Who am I? Finally, I'm beginning to open my eyes. How could I have been so blind?"*

Since Fabiana's heart and mind were opened, I continued. I explained to her how we create our own reality. Our perspective on who we are and how to live is distorted. Our five senses, which are our antennae, provide us only limited information. Through our eyes we see only colors from red to violet, but not infrared or ultraviolet. Our ears cannot pick up certain sounds that, for example, dogs do. When a tsunami or a hurricane is coming, animals sense something in the environment and run away to protect themselves. Most of us don't have that ability. We only perceive a portion of reality.

Taking off the masks of persona provides a chance to see the way we're actually living and feeling. We've been viewing our life from a single vantage point and acting as though that is all we are. As in the story of the blind people and the elephant (see chapter 2, "So ... What Is Cancer?"), **different people perceive the same situation differently.** It's as if we've gone through life wearing a pair of tinted glasses of a certain color and have seen everything only through that lens. When we meet someone wearing glasses like ours, we get along well. But when we encounter those who view the world differently, it can be difficult to find common ground. It's best to recognize that there are many ways of seeing life.

Our perspective becomes more complete when we integrate different points of view. Cover one eye and focus on an object, and then do the same with the other eye. What you see is slightly different with each eye. If we spent the rest of our life arguing which is correct, we'd lose the opportunity to discover the depth perception that binocular vision gives us.

"I understand that, under certain situations, it's important to take other points of view into account, but I don't understand what this has this to do with my health. I had cancer; that's a fact. There's no other way to look at it," Fabiana said.

No one was contesting that she'd had cancer (albeit in situ), I explained, but it can be important to see what cancer might mean in her life from other viewpoints. When faced with disease, we can **broaden our perspective and see in more depth what is happening to us.** Einstein said, *"No problem can be solved from the same level of consciousness that created it."* To "solve the problem," we need to explore the ground beneath the fact that a tumor invaded an organ and made us sick.

In chapter 2, "So ... What Is Cancer?," we saw how cancer can be the result of the way we adjust to internal and external events in our lives. How we respond to events is based on how we perceive them. For example, a person finds his workplace disturbing and not long after that is fired. From a certain level of consciousness, this dismissal is seen as a misfortune, and the person might be frightened by having to find a new job. This can lead to a state of vulnerability and possibly even illness. Another person might feel that life has granted her a favor in moving her from her upsetting workplace and respond to being fired with creativity and hope. **Our health-disease state is, at least in part, a manifestation of our perceptions and our attitude toward life.**

We saw in chapter 3, "Why Do We Get Sick?," that the way we perceive what's happening to us triggers thoughts, emotions, prejudices, wishes, labels, interpretations, judgments, dilemmas, memories, fears, certainties, beliefs, and hopes. Our perceptions express in our internal pharmacy through the PNIE network. Our consciousness isn't based solely on reality but also reflects our internal "settings." The critical variable is the information our consciousness uses to mold our body. Some people in stressful environments, e.g., develop skin rashes or welts. When our internal settings change, consciousness manifests it in the body, in this case on the skin.

People with multiple personality disorder show us how different levels of consciousness can result in different physical manifestations. A woman needed glasses with one personality and with another did not. A man was allergic to certain foods while in one personality, and in another he wasn't. **If we reset our consciousness, our body chemistry changes!**

"Okay, Laura, you've convinced me! I never thought that considering other points of view could be healing for me!" Fabiana said, her lips forming a smile. *"And to think, we spend so much time arguing about who's right, without getting anywhere."*

I agreed with Fabiana how polarized life is. We're either pro-this or anti-that; things are good or bad, known or unknown. We focus on polarities to navigate complexity.

Our brains have been trained to think in a linear way—effect follows cause. Reality is much more nuanced; seldom if ever, in nature and in life, do things happen in a linear way. **Faced with complexity, the mind doesn't know what to do and begins to classify things in one or another pole**—I like it, I don't like it; I agree, I disagree. We spend a lot of energy defending one pole. "This soccer team is better than that one," "That political party is better than this one," "Doing it this way is better than doing it that way."

To play soccer, it's helpful to recognize that we're part of a team. But remaining at that level of consciousness leads to confrontation, widening the gulf between one team and another, sometimes inciting violence. As Einstein suggests, if players would broaden their consciousness, they would understand that beyond team membership, the point is to play soccer wholeheartedly. Doing so, they align with the activity itself, enjoying the movement, exhilaration, task, and goal, without making the "other" wrong, bad, or the enemy, focusing instead on sport's entertainment value and opportunity for social connection.

We're at a moment in time when our minds are evolving from linear to complex thinking. If we were just linear, we could divide our bodies into parts—head, arms, torso, legs, then smaller parts—lungs, heart, aorta, vena cava, and even smaller until we reach the cellular level. Inversely, we could reassemble ourselves from cells to organs to body to human being. But it doesn't happen this way.

More than other diseases, cancer requires us to see ourselves as complex beings—body, mind, emotions, and spirit in a continuous, interactive dance. From the moment of diagnosis, cancer forces us to face a difficult situation. It's not like an infection, which can be easy to identify and treat with antibiotics. In the face of a cancer diagnosis, we rarely can point to a single, specific cause. Cancer is the outcome of multiple factors. It's an imbalance, a systemic failure wherein mind, body, and spirit have become disconnected, or fragmented. The way we relate inside and how we relate with others on the outside reflect each other. Cancer demands that we view the whole picture—external stresses, thinking, exercise, and nutrition. It requires that we look at our whole life to see what's out of balance. Cancer demands that we change our thinking from linear to complex.

How can we get out of the "duality trap"—healthy/sick, with cancer/without cancer, normal/abnormal lab results (cancer marker)? These are the patterns of linear thinking. Following Einstein, what would it be like to enter into complex thinking? **Healthy and sick are two sides of the same coin, two states of a being trying to express and unfold its essence.** Which would be the broadest level of consciousness that sees both sides of the coin and from that perspective seeks to find a holistic solution?

Fabiana returned the following week both open to what was new and, at the same time, overwhelmed. "Laura, it's all unfamiliar! I'm not used to living with this much uncertainty. Until now, my life has always followed a plan."

The only constant is change. It's been like this throughout the history of mankind. Today, however, change is occurring increasingly quickly. VUCA is an acronym coined by the American military; it stands for Volatile, Uncertain, Complex, and Ambiguous. This terminology has resonated with businesspeople as they try to make sense of the constantly changing challenges brought on by politics, economics, society, and the environment.

Cancer is an invitation to embark on a journey into the unknown. There's a lot to learn—medical terms, observing new sensations and mental reactions, fear, loss of control, uncertainty, and the possibility of death. Cancer's wake-up call can be compared to the beginning of the hero's journey.

The alarm clock rings and awakens us from the world of illusion. That alarm, or "call," may come as a crisis, a disease, a pain, or the feeling of not belonging, and it compels us to leave the routine of our life, often against our will. As protagonists in the hero's journey, we cannot ignore that call. If we ignore it, it will return again with ever more intensity.

The Hero's Journey

The hero's journey is a story repeated in many cultures and times, with different characters and locations, but always with the same message. The human being, at some time during his or her life, is called to enter a path of self-discovery. It's a difficult path into the hidden inner universe, in search of the treasure of the soul. By integrating the soul, the path leads to fulfillment.

This journey of initiation generally has three stages: the call or initiation, the departure (with transformative experiences), and the return.

In the *Odyssey,* Homer describes Odysseus's journey home to Ithaca after the Trojan War. It takes ten years, during which the hero faces unimaginable dangers. Facing these vicissitudes, he begins to discover himself. It is a journey of self-knowledge. Odysseus tells the cyclops Polyphemus that his name is "Nobody," suggesting that entering the transformative path requires not just getting away from one's familiar environment, but even his known identity, in order to experience renewal.

There are many examples of the hero's journey in literature and film: *Don Quixote, The Lord of the Rings,* and *Star Wars* are among them. *Finding Joe* is a documentary film about mythologist Joseph Campbell, who recognized the common theme of the hero's journey in cultures throughout the world.[1]

We must let go of the life we have planned, so as to accept the one that is waiting for us.
—Joseph Campbell

The hero's journey takes us on a road to the unknown, a road filled with challenges and adventures that sooner or later we all must face. There are no shortcuts. **The only way out is through.** The way to begin the journey is different for each of us, and our **attitude makes a difference.** Whether we venture forth with a positive or a negative attitude will affect the experience.

It's a journey of transformation. As we come to know ourselves better, enter new situations, and find new ways to connect with others, we're transformed by it. It's a journey to the universe inside of us. We won't see clearly where we're going, and we'll lose control. This road is part of life's mystery. Accepting and surrendering to our own inner voice is the way to be transformed.

"I understand everything you're telling me," Fabiana said. *"It all makes sense. But how is it accomplished?"*

I assured her she was on the right path. Becoming aware that this crisis demands a change and searching for an explanation beyond the physical diagnosis is the first step. **The path begins by becoming conscious of how we've been living,** how we've been taking care of ourselves, what thoughts and feelings we have, how we react and connect with others, the connection we have with what's important to us and gives meaning to our life.

Broadening our perspective helps integrate the parts inside us, even those that seem inconsistent with each other and with our sense of who we are. The integration of body, mind, and spirit helps us live a life of fulfillment, creating space around the pain that was taking all of our attention and instead creating a space where something new can be born.

During these first sessions, we tried to identify what had led Fabiana to this imbalance. It was essential she identify what was and what wasn't working for her. What could she learn from her present situation?

Giving the disease new meaning can help us abandon our sense of being a victim. Living consciously empowers us to change our focus toward what's important in life, to make decisions and changes to return to a healthy path. Since the path of self-knowledge integrates the soul, the decisions we make at this time can be inspired by the wishes of the soul. If the decisions keep coming from our mind, or ego, we'll probably continue, more or less, the same basic patterns. I emphasized to Fabiana that this was an adventure, like the adventures of heroes of old.

Assuming responsibility for her own health and committing to make necessary changes to return to a healthy path is the second stage. I told Fabiana she needed to prepare for a long journey. We went over how to fill in her energy tank (see chapter 5, "Energize Your Body!") to be ready. She needed to sustain her motivation and not succumb to fear.

There's no magical remedy to return to healthy living. There's not one formula that's useful for everyone. It depends on what the disease is trying to tell each person. Sometimes the message is to stop. That might be the case for someone experiencing too much stress at work. For someone with chronic sadness, not finding purpose in life, a healthy path might be to connect with what brings pleasure, what has energy, what is important and makes his or her heart sing.

The path I recommended to Fabiana wouldn't be easy for her. I suggested she seek and accept help. To facilitate change, **it's important to create favorable conditions and choose good company.** Don Quixote chose

Sancho Panza. In *Lord of the Rings,* Frodo chose his gardener and his friends Pippin and Merry. Good companions believe in the project of your growth and commit to it.

For Fabiana and others with cancer, it's important to see the disease as an opportunity to make needed changes, and they must be ready to find ways to support change, giving it their all. It's essential to surround yourself with positive family members, friends, and professionals.

The companion's role is to support—and not be a burden—for the sick person, not making demands about what must or must not be done. The one who makes decisions and chooses what's beneficial is the person himself or herself. The rest of the team is there to support and advise (when asked). People who see cancer as a "misfortune that fell from the sky" and want everything to return to "normal," the way it was before, are not good company. Returning to normal means recreating the conditions that led to getting sick.

The integrative physician's role is to support the person as he or she explores areas beyond the normal comfort zone to risk making changes. A good coach doesn't give answers but encourages the person to become aware, from the inside, so that person can find solutions consistent with internal values, choices, and perspective.

This requires a customized follow-up from the physician, who must have a genuine interest in guiding the person toward the best combination of treatments, therapies, and practices for restoring a healthy balance. The person must agree to participate actively and undertake the work of restoring his or her own health.

"What should I focus on?" Fabiana asked.

Our Actions Matter

We are what our thoughts have made us, so take care of what you think.

Words are secondary. Thoughts live; they travel far.

—Swami Vivekananda

Incorporating too many new ideas and exercises at the same time can be counterproductive. I suggested Fabiana give priority to what's most essential, which I believe is to focus on the **way of thinking that molds our life.** Thinking leads to attitude, which leads to lifestyle choices. An unhealthy lifestyle is largely responsible for the imbalances that lead to *dis-ease.* When we lack ease, at some point, the body will show it.

By changing our way of thinking we can achieve a healthier life.

Practice for Healthy Living

Choose your thoughts as if we were all telepaths and happy to hear to what you think.[2]

We are a walking pharmacy, producing our own internal medicines according to the way we live. If we change our thoughts, we can encourage our "internal pharmacist" to produce the substances that will make us healthy and stimulate our immune system. Attention must be focused on building our own energy and avoiding people and situations that harm or steal our energy.

"Yes, Laura, thanks! It's true I need to change my way of thinking. I let myself be carried away by fear-based thoughts, always focusing on the problem. If I could change my thoughts, I would win the battle!"

Fabiana was accepting that prioritizing thoughts is essential. And she was able to recognize how a change of thought shifts the paradigm in which we live.

Winning what battle, though? If cancer is a manifestation of our own body, who is Fabiana fighting against? Who is the enemy? Some part of herself? And if it's really a question of winning, who will the winner be? The person who lives the longest, even if he or she continues to live out of balance? Which is a better life—ninety-nine years regardless of quality, or thirty-three years in service to humankind?

The paradigm shift means changing the thought of cancer as an enemy to seeing it as a warning, a message to return to our unique and genuine path.

When we try to fit into the mold of life as others and our conditioning tell us it should be, we ignore or repress parts of ourselves, and eventually we'll get sick.

Health has to do with a balance of body, mind, and spirit. We are an open system in continuous dialogue with the environment and other people. A healthy being responds to what life presents. To stay healthy, it's important to maintain a permanent exchange—breathing, eating, excreting waste, relating with others, laughing, dancing, enjoying, and experimenting. A system that ceases to exchange, that closes itself off, fades out and goes toward death. To be healthy, it's essential to keep life pulsing.

In a complex system, when one part is modified, all the other parts are affected. When we start to exercise and eat healthy foods, the results can be more profound than anticipated. We might not only lose weight, but our heart will have less stress on it, our self-esteem might rise, and we'll connect again with what gives meaning to our life. Small changes in our system can have a large impact on our health. Medicine is not mathematics, which might explain in part the miraculous recoveries that sometimes occur.[3]

The seed has within it all the information needed to produce the tree, its flowers and fruits. But it can only germinate, grow, and blossom with the necessary conditions of temperature, humidity, and nutrition. If these conditions diminish, the plant might dry up. Like the seed, we have all the information we need in our essence. And to grow and blossom, we need adequate conditions. If life turns out difficult and we don't know how to respond to the conditions, we too might dry up.

Cancer is not leading us into battle, but to a creative exploration to discover what is hidden within, so we can lead a more conscious life expressing our fullest potential. The goal is not victory over another, not even victory over a disease, which we've established is simply a messenger, but to be able to offer the world and humankind our essence, the fragrance of the flower we are, the most creative and authentic person only we can offer.

Even death can be a wake-up call. Of course, we all want to get well, to recover fully from our illness. But waking up is more than even recovering. It is accepting who we are, being present for our unique life, staying present whatever we encounter. We can awaken, be conscious and filled with love, even with our last breath.

Waking up means to be aware, as the Buddhists say, of "things as they are," of whatever hand of cards we've been dealt. We do our utmost to regain our health, restore our balance, and feel as alive as we possibly can. We must not forget, illness can be an opportunity to step outside the image of who we or others think we're supposed to be and into our life as it is.

The purpose of life is to live, to express our soul's essence fully. It's not a matter of quantity but of quality. The purpose of a flower is to bloom, to display its splendor and share its fragrance. Just as a seed germinates, turns into a seedling, and then a plant, we can also unfurl and offer our unique beauty and wisdom. It makes no sense trying to be a rose if, in our essence, we are a dandelion.

"A bird doesn't sing because it has an answer, it sings because it has a song."[4] Even in the last moment of life, we can express completely who we are—not as an image, but as a person. We can wake up to health, to aliveness, to gratitude, and when the time comes, to dying. Some of us may only hear the call at the last moment. And even then, we have the chance to awaken.

No one knows better than you do what's good for you. And the best way to know is to stay connected with your body.

Let your body guide you.
The clues are inside of you.
You are your own authority.

What makes you feel alive? What fills you with excitement? What makes you feel truly happy? Take the path that leads in that direction.

Take-Home Message
Cancer invites us to wake up and transform ourselves.

The first step, a big one, is to dare answer the call and be open to change.

How can we face change?

• Become aware of how we're living.

• Take responsibility for our own health.

• Commit to change.

• Create the necessary conditions.

• Choose good company.

Attitude makes the difference.

Face crises with energy, optimism, and hope.

Our way of thinking molds our life.

Being healthy or sick are two sides of the same coin, two states of a being trying to find and express its essence.

There's no magical formula to finding a healthy path.

Small changes can make big differences.

The clues are inside you.

You can wake up and be yourself, no matter what.

EPILOGUE

The world is undergoing many levels of crises—political, educational, institutional, social, ethical, and familial. Crisis: is it a danger or an opportunity? Every crisis invites us to wake up, open our eyes, see the ways we're living, and choose patterns that support our well-being. Today's crises are, in fact, triggering a collective awakening.

It's strange that in other times and cultures, men and women considered waking up to who we are a priority, and they kept this alive through myths, legends, and initiation rites that inspire wholeness. In the twenty-first century, we no longer have rites of passage to usher us into a more awakened life.

Cancer is now one of the most frequently diagnosed diseases in the West, and incidences are increasing every year. What is this epidemic trying to tell us? Many of those going through the cancer experience are way-showers. Their explorations and learnings enrich us all.

We're starting to realize that the way we eat is unhealthy, and there's a food revolution challenging even our most basic habits. We're seeing that it's not worthwhile to spend our lives focused solely on working and making money, that it's better to find what makes us happy and devote our lives to that. We're starting to understand that emotions can make us sick, and that to stay healthy we need to be mindful of how we relate to others and value the loving ties we have. We've discovered that what keeps us well and truly alive is connecting with what gives our life meaning. Many who have gone through a cancer experience agree that with or without cancer, living an awakened life is best. It's not a coincidence that one of these people defines their cancer experience as "a gift, though a pity it comes in such ugly packaging."

Might cancer be our modern initiation rite? Is it possible that deep down we know there is a hidden treasure within us waiting to be discovered and shared with others? Can cancer be a wake-up call, a call to awaken to who we really are, to what we've come into the world to do and to be? Cancer can lead us to a transformative path, one difficult to travel without such extreme prodding. I hope you feel encouraged discovering this new way to look at cancer, not as an enemy or merely a physical disease, but as a guide that can encourage you on the most rewarding journey life has to offer.

Appendix 1

NUTRITION

Urban Legends

There's an abundance of advice on nutrition available in books, articles, online, and elsewhere. Some of it is helpful, while much is less well grounded. Let's analyze some of these urban legends.

It's necessary to become a vegetarian.

Vegetarian diets can be of great benefit for health. A vegetarian diet is based on leafy green and other vegetables, legumes, fruits, grains, and seeds, and it excludes animal products. There are different kinds of vegetarian diets:

- Vegan: a strict vegetarian diet that excludes all meat, dairy, eggs, and other animal products
- Lacto vegetarian diet: allows dairy products

- Ovo-lacto vegetarian diet: allows eggs and dairy products

Among these, the most important ones tend to be low in saturated fats and high in fiber, vitamins, and phytochemicals,[1] insofar as they exclude red and processed meats. For these reasons, vegetarian diets help reduce cancer risk. However, becoming a vegetarian is not necessary, since a diet low in consumption of red meats and animal fats offers similar results.

For those who follow a strict vegetarian diet, it's necessary to monitor the levels of vitamin B12, zinc, iron, and calcium, which can be scarce and affect health—for example, leading to anemia and bone fractures.

Natural products are better and aren't harmful.

In the aftermath of the processed food industry's boom, we realize that homemade foods are healthier than processed or refined ones. Unfortunately, we can't be sure what products labelled "natural" actually are, since labeling laws vary from country to country. In the US, the term *natural* means next to nothing.[2]

We also need to be cautious about supplements and natural herbs. Supplements advertised as "natural" are not always better or safer than refined or processed ones. Many plants and fruits, though natural, are toxic or fatal for our body when ingested—for example, hemlock. Mushrooms are also completely natural, but some are toxic, i.e., neither safe nor useful for humans. Natural foods and nutritional supplements may also be contaminated by fungi. Since these are removed during processing, in these cases, a manufactured product may be safer than a natural one.

If it's been used through the ages, it must be good.

Just because a substance might have been used in folk or traditional medicine doesn't mean it's safe and effective. It's true that if it were toxic, it would not have been tolerated and would no longer be used. However, substances used in traditional medicines are not studied rigorously, and they might, e.g., have long-term cumulative effects that have never been detected. Some folk remedies used today are no longer prepared as before or are used out of context, and their effect isn't the same as in days past. For example, there are herbs used in Peru to treat "fever." *Fever* in many places is a synonym for malaria, and the herbs are mainly anti-parasitic.[3] If one of these products is used in another place to treat a fever caused, e.g., by bacteria, it will not have the same result.

If it were harmful, it could not be sold.

The process of analysis and authorization of new medicines is much more rigorous than that of nutritional supplements. To be approved as a medicine, a substance must undergo strict tests regarding toxicology, interaction with other drugs, and use in individuals with different diseases, and it must be proven safe and efficient in different situations. These studies can take years and are expensive, which, in part, is why new medicines tend to be expensive.

The approval process for dietary supplements is less strict. For the most part, rigorous tests of safety and efficiency aren't conducted, and authorities generally only intervene if problems arise after they're available for sale. Thus, there may be products available that cause adverse effects as yet unknown.

If it's sold over the counter, it's not a medicine and cannot interfere with my prescription drugs.

For the same reason supplements are approved without rigorous analyses of safety and efficiency, or of interaction with medicines, there may be supplements available that have severe interactions with medicines, and this might be unknown (see "Vitamins and Supplements" in the glossary that follows). Some herbs interfere with medicines' metabolism or elimination, and as a consequence become toxic.

This is worse in the case of a strong medicine like chemotherapy, since toxicity can result in extreme symptoms, even death.

There are many examples of natural products that turned out to be toxic or interfered with oncological treatments, increasing their toxicity or reducing their efficiency. A recent example is green tea's interaction with bortezomib, a chemo drug used to treat multiple myeloma. Studies were conducted to see if green tea could increase bortezomib's efficiency, and surprisingly, they came to the opposite conclusion—that green tea reduces its activity. A similar result is that high amounts of antioxidants counteract the effects of many chemo drugs (see chapter 6, "From Treating Cancer to Treating the Whole Person").

For this reason, it's important to inform your physician about all herbs, supplements, and other substances you are taking or wish to take, especially if you're undergoing chemotherapy or another anticancer treatment.

If a small quantity is good, a larger quantity is better.

Since the 1990s, there has been a tendency to believe that megadoses of vitamins are beneficial, even though scientific studies do not support this idea.

Some minerals and vitamins in high doses may, in fact, have deleterious effects. Vitamins A, D, E, and K cannot easily be expelled from the body, and the consumption of high doses of these vitamins results in an accumulation that can be toxic. High doses of vitamin C interfere with the absorption of essential minerals such as copper, and high doses of phosphorus interfere with the absorption of calcium. In relation to cancer, studies of patients treated with chemo show that high doses of vitamins may interfere with chemotherapy's effects, making it less effective or more toxic (see chapter 6, "From Treating Cancer to Treating the Whole Person").

Glossary

Additives

IS IT TRUE THAT ADDITIVES AND PRESERVATIVES IN PACKAGED FOODS MIGHT CAUSE CANCER?

Many substances are added to foods during processing. Additives might be natural or synthetic (chemical) and are added to foods not for their nutritive value, but to prolong shelf and storage life and enhance appearance, taste, color, etc.

Authorized additives are classified according to their functions. The nomenclature system found on the labels of packaged foods throughout the world is that of the European Union, composed of numbers following the letter E, such as E-330, E-300, and E-950. In the US, additives are generally referred to by name rather than series number.

Additives Nomenclature

The International Numbering System for Food Additives (INS) is a European-based naming system for food additives aimed at providing a brief designation for what may be a lengthy actual name. It's defined by Codex Alimentarius, the food standards organization of the World Health Organization (WHO) and the Food and Agriculture Organization of the United Nations (FAO). This information is published in the document "Class Names and the International Numbering System for Food Additives," first published in 1989, revised in 2008 and 2011. The INS is an open list, "subject to the inclusion of additional additives or removal of existing ones on an ongoing basis."[4]

Series E-100–E-199 (colorants)	These add color to foods. Sometimes they're added to compensate for the loss of color that takes place during food processing. At other times, they're used to boost sales, since a product's color can lead consumers to select it.
Series E-200–E-299 (preservatives)	These are used to delay a food's degradation, preventing the development of yeast and bacteria (microorganisms).
Series E-300–E-399 (antioxidants)	These help food stay in good condition and prevent fats from becoming rancid.

Series E-400–E-499 (agents affecting texture: stabilizers, thickeners, emulsifiers, and gels)	These are mainly used to stabilize fat-and-water combinations, emulsions such as margarine, mayonnaise, and salad dressing. The ones used most are E-322 (soy lecithin), E-471, and E-472.
Series E-500–E-599 (acidity (pH) regulators, anti-caking agents)	These additives have different functions. Some regulate acidity to better preserve foods; others prevent caking and agglomeration in flour products.
Series E-600–E-699 (flavor enhancers)	These are flavor enhancers. The best known is monosodium glutamate (MSG) or E-621, used frequently in Asian cooking. It's also known as the umami additive. Umami (savory) is one of the five basic tastes, along with bitterness, sweetness, sourness, and saltiness, and is found naturally in some foods such as meat, spinach, and mushrooms. MSG is produced by a chemical process, and eating it, for some people, produces dizziness, illness, sweating, weakness, tachycardia, or breast pain, among other symptoms. Since MSG functions as a neurotoxin affecting the nervous system's cells, its consumption should be avoided, especially by children.

Series E-900–E-999 (various)	These include sweeteners used in low-calorie products, substances without nutritional value that give food a sweet taste. The best known are acesulfame-K (E-950), aspartame (E-951), isomaltitol (E-953), saccharin (E-954), and xylitol (E-967). This series also includes glazing agents, such as beeswax (E-901), used to cover certain foods.

Some additives are nutrients, for example, vitamins C and E, which are sometimes added to food products as preservatives. But most additives lack nutritional value and may cause adverse effects, such as those experienced when consuming MSG.

Some additives are said to be carcinogens or precursors of carcinogens. The most controversial ones include sodium nitrates and nitrites, cyclamate, and saccharin. Adverse effects of additives, especially cancer risk, are a matter of great public concern.

Studies show that in large quantities (more than is used in food products), some additives might cause cancer in animals. However, in food products additives are usually present in small quantities. The maximum daily intake of these substances that can be consumed without representing a significant risk for human health has been defined and can be found in the database of the Joint FAO/WHO Expert Committee on Food Additives (JECFA).[5] Food additives are strictly regulated. Before being approved for use by each country's authorities, additives must undergo exhaustive studies to guarantee their safety, especially to eliminate cancer risk.

Although the use of particular additives in acceptable doses should not cause major harm, the accumulation of various additives, even in small amounts, can overload our organism, in particular those organs responsible for metabolism and elimination. This affects the PNIE network, disturbing its operation and making it less efficient. A PNIE network imbalance increases our vulnerability to disease, including cancer.

CAN FOODS CONTAIN SUBSTANCES NOT INCLUDED ON THEIR LABELS?

In addition to additives that have been approved for use (in some countries, these must be included on labels), foods also contain *polluting elements* that reach consumers unnoticed.

Chemical compounds used in agriculture, in animal-breeding centers, in processing or packaging, or in the air or ocean water, find their way onto and into foods—even those not intended for human consumption. Examples include hormones and antibodies used in animal farming, small amounts of pesticides and herbicides in plant-based foods, compounds such as bisphenol A (BPA) that enter food from packaging, and heavy metals, such as cadmium and mercury, that accumulate in fish.

Unintended contamination of foods can result in exposure to chemicals that are of concern and may be related to the risk of cancer. Some of these compounds are not known to directly cause cancer, but they may influence cancer risk in other ways, such as BPA, which interferes with hormonal cycles.[6]

Algae and Spirulina

I'VE BEEN TOLD ALGAE ARE GOOD. CAN I INCLUDE THEM IN MY DIET?

Algae are a rich food source. They contain vitamins, minerals, and antioxidants. Among them, spirulina,[7] blue-green algae, is one of the favorites because it's easily digested and rich in proteins.

Due to its high content of proteins and essential amino acids (those we cannot produce and must include in our diet), spirulina is a beneficial complement to vegetarian diets. It is usually regarded as a supplement rather than a protein replacement, because large amounts need to be consumed to provide the daily requirement of proteins.

Due to its iron content, its consumption is recommended in cases of iron deficiency anemia.[8] It also provides other minerals, such as manganese, copper, zinc, and selenium.

It contains vitamins, such as vitamin A or carotenoids, complex B vitamins (including B12, important for vegetarians), and vitamin E. It also provides antioxidants and linoleic acid, which is not usually included in daily diets and promotes heart and joint health.

Studies suggest that spirulina may stimulate the immune system, but this has not yet been demonstrated in human beings.[9]

Spirulina can be taken in powder or tablets. The daily recommended dose to keep healthy is 500mg. Before taking spirulina daily, some preventive measures need to be considered:

- Since spirulina may have a stimulant effect on the immune system, it could be beneficial for a person with infection or with cancer, but not for someone with an autoimmune disease.
- It could also interfere with medications used as immunosuppressants in these diseases and with methotrexate chemotherapy, used in breast cancer treatment. Since it also

interacts within the metabolism of many medications (e.g., cytochrome P450), it could increase the toxicity of other medications or inhibit their effect. People receiving chemotherapy or other medications should consult their physician before taking spirulina.

- Since spirulina is rich in all amino acids, including phenylalanine, people suffering from phenylketonuria should not consume it.
- The iodine content of spirulina varies greatly, depending on how it was raised. Since spirulina *may* be rich in iodine, it should be *consumed with caution in hyperthyroidism* conditions, including Hashimoto's disease, to avoid stimulating the thyroid even more. In areas lacking iodine, foods or salt are often fortified to guarantee that the local population receives the minimal recommended dose of iodine. If this element needs to be supplemented even more, for example for those suffering from

iodine deficiency or hypothyroidism, spirulina might be a good option.

- Algae are nourished by water and sun and may be polluted by toxic substances (e.g., microcystin, that causes damage to the kidneys and liver and toxicity in the nervous system) and by heavy metals found in water. It's important to look for organic algae or algae grown in a place that is guaranteed not to be polluted.
- Caution should be taken, as too much iodine adversely affects the thyroid. People receiving medications for thyroid disorders must consult their physicians to know if they can take spirulina, or if they need to adjust their levothyroxine dose before modifying their diet.

Alkalize Your Diet

HOW DOES AN ALKALINE DIET WORK?

As we saw in chapter 5, "Energize Your Body!," normal cells must be in slightly alkaline conditions to function well.

A diet rich in acidic foods, with few alkalizing foods or basis, will force the organism to work hard to keep the pH slightly alkaline. When there is a lack of alkalizing foods or an excess of acidic foods, the body must compensate for the acidification.

There are two ways to compensate: deposit the acidic excess in the body (rheumatism, circulatory disorders) or remove the alkaline reservoir in the body (calcium, magnesium, potassium) deposited in bones, joints, teeth, and nails. That is why acidifying foods demineralize the organism, make bones more fragile, and promote the development of osteoporosis.

Following are two lists of foods, the first showing which ones contribute to alkalinity and are recommended, the second showing which are acidifying and should be reduced or removed from your diet.

Alkalizing foods (healthy and beneficial)

- All raw vegetables. Although some raw vegetables are acidic, they produce alkalinization within the organism. Others are slightly acidifying but provide the minerals acting as bases[10] or alkaline substances. When cooked, many vegetables have acidifying effects.

- Fruits. Lemon has a very acid pH (approximately 2.2), but within the organism it has an alkalizing effect. Drinking the juice of one lemon (in a liter of water) every day is recommended.
- Seeds and nuts. Almonds, for example, are highly alkalizing.
- Whole-grain cereals. Millet is alkalizing; others are slightly acidifying, but very healthy. They must be whole-grain and be cooked.
- Plant chlorophyll. Highly alkalizing.
- Sodium bicarbonate, commonly known as baking soda, weakly ionizes in water. One-quarter teaspoon of sodium bicarbonate may be taken in half a glass of water in the morning and before getting into bed, as a supplement.

Foods that acidify the organism (unhealthy)

- Refined sugar and all products containing it
- Meats in general
- Cow's milk and its byproducts
- Refined salt
- Refined flour and all products containing it: pasta, pizza, pastries, breads (which are also unhealthy since most contain saturated fats, margarine, salt, sugar, and preservatives)
- Margarine
- Soft drinks
- Caffeine
- Alcohol
- Any cooked food (cooking removes oxygen and turns it into acid), even cooked vegetables
- Packaged foods (contain preservatives, colorants, flavor enhancers, stabilizers)
- Other substances, like tobacco and medications including chemotherapy

Antioxidants and Phytochemicals

WHAT ARE ANTIOXIDANTS, AND HOW DO THEY RELATE TO CANCER?

An **antioxidant** is a molecule that inhibits free radicals, which are highly reactive, unstable molecules that can cause damage to parts of cells such as proteins, DNA, and cell membranes by stealing their electrons through a process called oxidation. Although we're not aware of it, antioxidants and free radicals are permanently fighting a battle inside of us.

Normal processes of our organism produce free radicals, and our immune system uses them, e.g., to kill germs and viruses. We're also exposed to environmental factors that produce free radicals, such as industrial pollutants, cigarette smoke, radiation, certain medicines, chemical additives in processed foods, and pesticides.

When we're exposed to large amounts of free radicals or if their production in us gets out of control and their numbers exceed those of antioxidants, problems arise. When free radicals are no longer held in check by antioxidants, a chain reaction is triggered, and oxidative stress arises. Molecules critical for cells to be kept alive and function properly are damaged, and they might injure and even kill healthy cells or produce cancer cells. Antioxidants can terminate these chain reactions by removing free radical intermediates and inhibit other oxidation reactions. They do this by being oxidized themselves, so antioxidants are often reducing agents such as thiols, ascorbic acid, or polyphenols.

Since oxidative stress has been associated with the pathogenesis of many human diseases, antioxidant use is being studied intensively to treat strokes and neurodegenerative diseases. Antioxidants are also widely used in dietary supplements in the hope of maintaining good health and preventing cancer and ischemic cardiovascular diseases. While some studies suggest that antioxidant supplements are beneficial for health, other clinical trials have not identified any advantage for the tested formulations and that an excess of supplements can be harmful. In addition to these applications in medicine, antioxidants are widely used in industry, e.g., to preserve foods and cosmetics and prevent rubber and gasoline deterioration.

To understand the way antioxidants function, think of how adults are stable when they're in a relationship. If a person loses her partner, she becomes like a free radical searching for a new partner. The new partner may be single, or perhaps someone else's partner. In the latter case, this sets off a chain reaction. New couples are formed to the detriment of others that become separated.

Antioxidants are like matchmakers, introducing free electrons to form couples and, in so doing, stabilizing free radicals and stopping the chain reaction. Just as matchmakers provide stability to a community, antioxidants delay or prevent the deterioration or oxidation[11] of other molecules when they neutralize free radicals.

We saw in chapter 5, "Energize Your Body!," that a healthy diet with fruits and vegetables provides us with the antioxidants used by plants to prevent their own deterioration.[12] Among antioxidants, we find vitamin C, vitamin E, vitamin A, resveratrol, and many other phytochemicals. Some fruits, for example citrus and red fruits, and vegetables like cauliflower, broccoli, eggplant, garlic, onions, and parsley, are rich in antioxidants. We can also find antioxidants in olives, ginger, turmeric, green tea, and chocolate.

Research shows that people who eat more fruits and vegetables may have a lower risk of developing certain kinds of cancer. But this does not necessarily mean that antioxidants are responsible for the result, because fruits and vegetables have many other compounds as well. In fact, studies that used antioxidant supplements (not whole fruits and vegetables) did not show a reduction in the risk of cancer. Many even reported an increase in cancer risk (see chapter 6, "From Treating Cancer to Treating the Whole Person"). High doses of beta-carotene and/or vitamin A in the form of supplements, for example, were shown to increase (not reduce) the risk of lung cancer among smokers. The best current advice for reducing the risk of developing cancer is to **get antioxidants directly from fruits and vegetables rather than from multivitamin supplements.**

There's evidence that antioxidants may improve the effects of chemo or radiation therapy,[13] but other research shows the opposite—that antioxidants can interfere with chemo or radiation. Considering the controversy, it's advisable to avoid taking high doses of antioxidants during chemotherapy and/or radiation as it might interfere with the effectiveness of the treatment. It would be unfortunate to bear the adverse side effects of chemotherapy, while at the same time, undermining its effectiveness. The decision whether or not to take antioxidants and at what dosage must be made by the person with his or her doctor, taking into account the person's characteristics, intention, kind of treatment, and the risk of side effects.

WHAT ARE PHYTOCHEMICALS, AND HOW CAN THEY REDUCE CANCER RISK?

Phytochemicals are biologically active compounds found in plants. Some of these compounds protect the plants against insects or have other essential functions. Many have antioxidant effects (see the entry above) or act as hormones, both in plants and in those who consume them. Considering that eating fruits and vegetables has been associated with a reduction of cancer risk, researchers have been trying to identify specific components responsible for this effect. There is currently no evidence that phytochemicals taken as supplements are as beneficial in the long term as those obtained from eating fruits, vegetables, fava beans, and grains.

Among phytochemicals, we can find flavonoids (found in soy, garbanzo beans, and tea), carotenoids (butternut squash, melons, and carrots are good sources), anthocyanins (responsible for the color of eggplants and red cabbage), and sulfites (found in garlic and onions).

Calcium

IS CALCIUM RELATED TO CANCER?

Many research studies suggest that food rich in calcium might reduce colorectal cancer, and that the consumption of calcium supplements reduces the recurrence of polyps. But a high consumption of calcium, whether through supplements or food, is also related to an increased risk of prostate cancer.

The situation of men is different from that of women. Considering the possible increase of prostate cancer with high levels of calcium, men should take the recommended daily dose but not exceed it. Women who show a higher risk of developing osteoporosis should try to achieve the recommended levels mainly through food intake and resort to dietary supplements only if necessary.

Green vegetables like spinach, broccoli, and watercress; nuts and seeds, such as hazelnuts, almonds, peanuts, pistachios, sunflower, and sesame seeds; raisins; figs; olives; parsley; cabbage; and legumes such as garbanzo beans, green beans, and other beans are excellent sources of calcium. In some cultures, people add crushed eggshells to food as a calcium supplement. You can also make sesame milk from sesame seeds.

How to Make Sesame Milk

Grind 1/4 cup of sesame seeds using a mortar or a grinder.

Blend the sesame with 1/2 liter (1 pint) of water.

Let it soften for four hours.

Strain using a mesh strainer, and it's ready to drink.

It's advisable to maintain appropriate levels of vitamin D to ensure good calcium absorption and metabolism.

Calcium can also be obtained from milk or dairy products. It would be convenient to choose low-fat or nonfat products to reduce the consumption of saturated fats (see "Milk and Dairy Products" in this glossary).

Recommended levels of calcium are 1,000 milligrams per day for people between nineteen and fifty years of age, and 1,200 milligrams per day for those fifty and older. For most people, 2.5 grams of calcium per day is safe, adding up the calcium in food, supplements, and antacids that contain calcium carbonate or sodium bicarbonate. Consuming higher doses of calcium might cause the formation of uric acid kidney stones, hypercalcemia, and kidney failure.

Coffee

DOES DRINKING COFFEE CAUSE CANCER?

There's no evidence that coffee or caffeine increases the risk of cancer. On the contrary, there's evidence that coffee might reduce the risk of skin cancer.[14]

Coffee is a stimulant and as such compels the body to be more active, even when we need a rest. It puts the body on alert, with a tendency to store everything we take in, therefore stimulating weight gain. In the middle of the day, when we feel exhausted from work, my advice is to take a break and practice relaxation for five or ten minutes, rather than drink coffee.

Colorants and Preservatives

See "Antioxidants and Phytochemicals."

Cooking

HOW DOES COOKING AFFECT THE RISK OF CANCER?

Cooking or heating vegetables breaks down vegetable cell walls, allowing for better digestion of the useful compounds. Many forms of food processing, such as freezing or canning of fruits and vegetables, may retain vitamins and other beneficial components. But many methods may also reduce the contents of some vitamins that are sensitive to heat, e.g., vitamin C,[15] the decrease of which might increase the risk of cancer. This is why it's advisable to eat a good portion of raw vegetables (see chapter 5, "Energize Your Body!").

It is necessary to cook meat well to kill dangerous microorganisms. Some studies, however, show that when frying, roasting, or grilling meat at very high temperatures, a chemical substance is produced (polycyclic aromatic hydrocarbons or heterocyclic aromatic amines) that might increase the risk of cancer. Slow simmering, steaming, boiling, and stewing are advisable, since they produce lower amounts of these chemicals.

Fats

DO WE NEED FATS? WHAT ARE GOOD FATS?

We need some fats, since many parts of the body have fat—such as the membrane covering each cell and the myelin sheath covering each neuron, allowing for the circulation of information through the nervous-system circuits. In addition, we get energy from fats for our daily activities. But eating fats in excess and eating low-quality fats are harmful.[16]

Fats are formed by units called fatty acids, linked like railroad cars to form saturated and unsaturated fats according to the predominant kind. Saturated fats increase low-density lipoprotein (LDL) cholesterol ("bad cholesterol"), which increases the likelihood of cardiovascular disease and strokes. This is why the intake of animal fats should be limited, since they're rich in saturated fats. Unsaturated fats help reduce LDL and are found in most vegetable oils, which are liquid at room temperature, such as olive oil, sunflower oil, and corn oil.

In urban areas, the average diet is far from healthy. We eat fats in excess, and even if we try to eat healthily, it's difficult, since many products have low-quality fats. When we eat animals raised on factory farms, for example, we consume saturated fats poor in omega-3 (see "Omega-3 and-6" in this glossary). Even many vegetable oils are hydrogenated to make them more stable at room temperature, and this promotes the formation of hydrogenated fats or trans fats (see "Do trans fats increase the risk of cancer?" below). Trans fats and omega-6 fatty acids are pro-inflammatory, which can be dangerous for the heart and associated with a higher risk of developing some kinds of cancer.

Reading nutritional information on labels helps you know the kinds and amounts of fats a product has.

DO TRANS FATS INCREASE THE RISK OF CANCER?

Trans fats are produced when vegetable oils are hydrogenated to produce oils like margarine or butter, which remain solid at room temperature. Trans fats raise levels of LDL cholesterol and reduce levels of high-density lipoprotein (HDL, or "good cholesterol") in blood, and therefore increase the risk of heart disease. It's advisable to limit or avoid the intake of trans fats, in light of their effect on the risk of heart disease.

One study showed that those who eat large amounts of trans fats have more oxidative stress and more free radicals in their urine, increasing the risk of cancer, particularly those who did not also eat antioxidant foods.

Trans fats are one of the least healthy foods, and the only way to avoid them is to avoid processed foods and margarine. Trans fats are used in many restaurants. If you limit your consumption of dairy products generally, it's better to consume butter than margarine. And it's always better to use olive oil or coconut oil than hydrogenated oils.

Fish

IS EATING FISH PROTECTION AGAINST CANCER?

Fish is a rich source of omega-3 fatty acids (see "Omega-3 and-6," in this glossary), and its consumption is associated with a reduced risk of heart disease. But fish quality is also important.

Some kinds of fish, particularly cold water and/or deep water fish, for example tuna and swordfish, may have high levels of polluting substances such as mercury and dioxins. Farm-raised fish are fed an artificial diet, and the fats of these fish are of a low quality. The fats we ingest are used to form our own fats (see "Fats" in this glossary), so it's important that we choose fats of a high quality.

It's advisable to eat wild-caught fish, since wild fish eat other fish and seafood. It's also advisable to rotate the kinds of fish you eat, to reduce exposure to the same toxins.[17]

Food Combining

HOW WE COMBINE FOODS IS IMPORTANT.

In addition to eating healthy foods in a calm atmosphere, chewing carefully, and being mindful, we should note that different foods have different requirements for optimal digestion. Depending on its texture (coarse or smooth, e.g., raw celery versus pureed celery) and its sugar, protein, and fat content, it is digested more quickly or slowly and in different areas of the digestive tract. Combining items with similar digestive requirements makes the process flow smoothly and helps the body receive maximum nourishment.

Combining items with different requirements can make digestion slower and less efficient.

Improper food combining can cause gas, heartburn, and an upset stomach. The two main rules of food combining to ensure efficient digestion and nutrition are:

- Don't eat proteins and starches at the same meal. This means no bun with your hamburger, no meatballs with pasta, no potatoes with meat.

- Don't eat fruits and vegetables at the same meal. Eat fruit thirty to sixty minutes before dinner.[18]

Genetically Modified Foods

WHAT ARE GENETICALLY MODIFIED FOODS? CAN THEY BE CONSUMED WITHOUT RISK?

Genetically modified organisms (GMOs) are plants, animals, and the products derived from them in which the deoxyribonucleic acid (DNA)[19] has been artificially altered through genetic engineering. They are created by adding genes from other plants or other organisms to obtain particular benefits, such as making them more resistant to insects, slowing down their decomposition, enhancing their flavors, increasing their nutritional content, or to acquire qualities they don't otherwise have.

Food manufacturers today resort more and more to genetic engineering. In the US, for example, a large proportion of soy is obtained from seeds that have been altered to resist herbicides; most of the corn is grown from seeds altered so that the corn itself produces an insecticide, as are many tomatoes and carrots. Thus, many food products manufactured with corn, soy, cotton, or canola include GMO crops among their ingredients.

Genetic modification could contribute to public health. For example, there's interest in increasing the folate content of some vegetables through genetic alteration. But many have doubts about GMO foods' safety. The added genes could produce substances that have negative consequences for consumers, such as allergic reactions, increased food intolerance, additional resistance to antibiotics, immune system suppression, or increased risk of cancer.

There's no hard evidence that genetically modified, commercialized foods are harmful for human health or might increase or reduce the risk of cancer. This lack of evidence doesn't necessarily imply the opposite, that they're safe. Genetically altered foods have been available only recently, and their long-term effects on human health are still unknown. To guarantee that consuming these foods is absolutely safe, their long-term effects must be evaluated. Only then can ingesting GMO foods be considered reliable and safe.

Ginger

WHAT IS GINGER USEFUL FOR?

Gingerroot has multiple properties. It relieves nausea and upset stomachs, reduces cholesterol, stimulates the immune system, and has antiinflammatory and analgesic (pain-relieving) properties. Several studies show that it inhibits the growth of cancer cells. The use of ginger is recommended for those under chemotherapy, to relieve nausea and vomiting.

It can be used in a variety of forms, including adding it to raw or cooked foods or desserts, or preparing ginger tea by adding small pieces of ginger to hot water.

Herbs

WHICH HERBS ARE BENEFICIAL FOR ME?

Supplements such as garlic, ginger, ginkgo biloba, and echinacea derive from plants and are sold as *natural* products. We've already seen (in "Natural products are better and aren't harmful" under "Urban Legends" at the beginning of this appendix) that natural doesn't necessarily mean harmless. Plants, herbs, and weeds contain many chemical substances, some of which are beneficial, while others are toxic or may cause allergies. In addition, sometimes these products are contaminated with fungi, toxic bacteria, pesticides, or heavy metals, all of which are deleterious for health.

Herbs and weeds derive from plants formed by roots, stems, leaves, and flowers, and each part may produce different effects in humans. For example, dandelion root provides a stimulating effect on the bowels, while its leaves produce a diuretic effect.[20] The effects of herbs depend on the dose. An infusion of a root or a leaf may produce beneficial effects, but the extract marketed in mother tinctures or pills might be in excessive doses.[21]

It's important to get reliable information about herbs and weeds before taking them, and to obtain them from sources that ensure their highest quality.

Irradiation

See "Processed Foods."

Juices

IS JUICING RECOMMENDED?

Drinking fruits and vegetables as shakes or juices may be a good way of ingesting them, especially if there are problems with chewing or swallowing. But juices have less fiber and might not give the same satisfaction as eating a whole fruit or vegetable.

Fruit and vegetable extracts aren't recommended, because they don't have healthy fiber, which helps with regularity. They act as prebiotics to feed the colon bacteria that help with digestion, and they allow sugar to be absorbed slowly, avoiding harmful sugar peaks. Extracts are basically natural juice with sugar, and when we drink them, they produce a sugar peak in blood and raise insulin (see "Sugar" in this glossary).

Fruit juices and shakes may contribute a large number of calories, particularly if you drink them in large quantities. It's better to prepare them at home or purchase products that have 100 percent fruits and vegetables and have been pasteurized to remove bacteria.

Milk and Dairy Products

CAN I DRINK MILK AND EAT DAIRY PRODUCTS?

Dairy products are one of the more contentious issues regarding a healthy diet. Studies on dairy products and their relation to the risk of cancer have had inconsistent results. Furthermore, the discussion of which elements in milk may be harmful—saturated fats, calcium, hormones, or a combination of them—has also been inconclusive. The Healthy Eating Plate, created by Harvard School of Public Health, provides detailed guidance to help us make the best eating choices. Their most recent version proposes reducing consumption of milk and dairy products to one or two portions a day.[22]

We've already advised reducing the consumption of saturated animal fats. In the case of milk and dairy products, you can choose low-fat or skim products, which have a lower fat content.

Regarding calcium in dairy products, studies have found that calcium reduces the risk of colon cancer. Other research shows that calcium increases the risk of prostate and ovarian cancer. Results are less convincing with regard to breast cancer. Many researchers think that, notwithstanding their calcium content, dairy products may cause osteoporosis[23] due to their high protein content, which acidifies the media[24] and promotes the reabsorption of calcium in the bones to counterbalance the acidity, producing bone weakening. But there isn't much scientific evidence to support this hypothesis. Most studies show that milk consumption increases bone health.

The breed of cows where milk comes from may be important. Milk with a certain subtype of milk protein or A1 beta-casein, the most common type found in cow's milk in Europe (excluding France), the US, Australia, and New Zealand, may be detrimental to health. However, A2-beta-casein milk, produced mostly by Guernsey cows, might not have such a deleterious effect. There are some companies in New Zealand producing A2 milk.

The milk we consume nowadays, obtained through mass production, is enriched with an estrogen derivative that might increase hormone-dependent cancer incidence, for example testicular, prostate, or breast cancer. Milk produced on farms where the cows' natural cycles are respected show less adverse effects on health.

It's advisable to limit the consumption of dairy products and take some precautions until their influence is clearer. We can get most of our calcium requirements from leafy green vegetables, legumes, and seeds (see "Calcium" in this glossary). If we consume dairy products, we can do so to a limited extent and choose low-fat or skimmed products.

Omega-3 and-6

MY FRIEND TAKES OMEGA-3 SUPPLEMENTS. SHOULD I DO THE SAME?

Each cell of our body is formed by fats that are formed by omega-3,-6, and-9 units. Picture a train that has some cars made of omega-3, some of omega-6, and some of omega-9. For the train to run smoothly, it needs a proper balance of the three materials. When these three kinds of fats are in proper proportions within a cell, the cell functions normally.

In the West, we often eat foods high in omega-6 and-9, but low in omega-3 fats. The ideal proportion is one omega-6 fat for each omega-3 fat. When the omega-6/omega-3 ratio is 20:1 or 50:1, which happens today, a person's health is threatened, including an increased risk of cancer. An imbalance in omega-6 and-3 fats is brought about by the foods we eat and the foods eaten by the animals we consume (see "Fats" in this glossary). To reverse this imbalance, we need to limit the consumption of omega-6 fats and take omega-3 supplements.

The main sources of omega-6 are common vegetable oils (corn, soy, canola, safflower, and sunflower oils). Their consumption should be limited especially in cooking because high temperatures facilitate the formation of trans fats (see "Do trans fats increase the risk of cancer?" in this glossary).

Omega-3 fats are found in walnut oil, flaxseed oil, flaxseeds, chia seeds, hemp, and other foods. The most beneficial form of omega-3 fatty acids is found only in fish and krill. To reach the recommended daily dose, large servings of fish should be consumed (e.g., 2.2 pounds of salmon per day). Since our diet, in general, lacks omega-3, and, since it's difficult to ingest two-plus pounds of salmon a day or the equivalent, the suggestion is to take fish oil or chia seed supplements (1,000mg per day).

Organic Foods

WHAT ARE ORGANIC FOODS?

The word *organic* is widely used to describe food products of vegetable or animal origin that do not use chemical substances, hormones, or antibiotics during their production. This classification does not include genetically modified or irradiated food products. Organic foods usually have an identifying label.

Organic foods are healthier for us because they don't contain chemicals (such as pesticides), hormones, or antibiotics that may affect health and overload our immune systems. There is not yet evidence that organic foods are more effective in reducing the risk of cancer. Some studies suggest that they have a higher nutritional content, while others suggest that there's no significant difference when they are compared with similar foods produced by conventional methods.[25]

Considering that this matter is not at all clear, whenever possible, it's better to choose organic foods. Whether or not they are organic, it's important to include vegetables, fruits, and grains in your diet.

WHAT IF I CAN'T GET ORGANIC FOODS?

Most pesticides, waxes, colorants, and other substances added to fruits, vegetables, and legumes reside on the skin, so it's wise to peel them when possible. If they can't be peeled, as in the case of strawberries, lettuce, or green beans, it's recommended to wash them carefully.

- To remove pesticide residues from food products, the first step is washing.
- About 75 to 80 percent of pesticide residues are removed by cold-water washing. Pesticide residues on the surface of fruits like grapes, apples, guava, plums, mangoes, peaches, and pears, as well as fruity vegetables like tomatoes, eggplant, and okra, require *two to three washings.*
- Washing with *2 percent saltwater* will remove most pesticide residues that normally appear on the surfaces of vegetables and fruits.

Fill a sink or container with lukewarm water, measuring the number of cups. Add one teaspoon of sea salt for every cup of water. Stir, place fruits and vegetables in the solution, and let them soak. After a few minutes, remove them and rinse with fresh water.

- Leafy green vegetables must be washed thoroughly. Pesticide residues from leafy green vegetables are normally removed by washing, blanching, and cooking.[26]

Pesticides

DO PESTICIDES AND HERBICIDES CONTAINED IN FOODS CAUSE CANCER?

Many pesticides are carcinogenic,[27] and most have not even been studied exhaustively to evaluate their effects on human beings. Pesticides and herbicides may be toxic when a person is directly exposed to them without protection in industrial or agricultural facilities. They reach the public, even in very low doses, through fruits and vegetables. Nowadays, pesticides and herbicides also reach human beings through water. Since they are used on crops and also in gardens, parks, and golf courses, after rains the runoff finds its way into streams, lakes, and rivers and contaminates our water sources.

At present, there is no evidence suggesting that residues of pesticides and herbicides in the low doses contained in foods increase cancer risk in humans. But pesticides build up in our body, and since the body cannot eliminate them, they affect our PNIE network. They could increase allergies, fertility problems, and diseases, including cancer. Therefore, it is advisable to consume organic fruits and vegetables whenever possible and to wash them thoroughly before eating (see "Organic Foods" in this glossary).

Processed Foods

IS IT TRUE THAT PROCESSED FOODS ARE MAKING US SICK?

In the last decades, processed foods have invaded our homes because they're easy to use and last for a long time (due to preservatives). They are not innocuous. Many contain salt, sugar, and fats that are added to make them tastier and more addictive. They activate the same areas of the brain stimulated by cocaine, and induce us to increase our intake and gain weight, which has serious consequences.

Foods may be altered during their processing, and this may increase the cancer risk. For example, when grains are refined, a large amount of fiber and other compounds that may reduce cancer risk are lost. Before being processed, some foods must be cooked, and this may remove vitamins and nutritive substances that reduce the risk of cancer (see "Cooking" in this glossary).

"IF IT WERE GOOD, IT'D BE GROWING FROM TREES."[28]

Here are some of the ways processed foods affect our health:

- They're addictive and lead to weight gain.
- The additives increase the risk of allergies and other diseases, such as cancer.

- Since they're poor in nutrients, they adversely affect our health. Sometimes vitamins and minerals are added to processed foods to compensate for the lack of nutrients, but these can never be compared to natural foods prepared at home. Plants and animals we consume have thousands of nutrients that are essential for good health, some in low amounts that science is just beginning to detect.
- They are low in fiber. White rice and refined flour are examples of processed foods that are much less healthy than their whole grain versions.
- Since they're normally digested more quickly than non-processed foods, they require less energy expenditure, which leads to weight gain.
- They contain refined sugar and fructose (see "Sugar" in this glossary), which lead to an increase of glycemia, insulin-dependency, and metabolic syndrome.
- They contain additives, including chemical sweeteners that are

carcinogenic, and taste enhancers, such as MSG, which have adverse effects on health (see "Additives" in this glossary).

- They contain nitrates and nitrites to preserve meat (sausage, bacon, and cold cuts), which are transformed in the stomach into' nitrosamines, which are carcinogenic.
- They contain caffeine, which increases the risk of osteoporosis, because it is an acidifying substance.
- They contain inexpensive fats, including hydrogenated ones that produce trans fats (in margarine and manufactured bakery products), associated with cardiovascular disease and some types of cancer (see chapter 5, "Energize Your Body!").
- They contain an imbalance between omega-3 and omega-6 (see "Omega-3 and-6" in this glossary) with an increase of omega-6—which favors inflammation, oxidation, and the production of free radicals (see "Antioxidants and Phytochemicals" in this glossary).

- They contain pesticides (see "Pesticides" in this glossary).
- They contain genetically modified organisms (see "Genetically Modified Foods" in this glossary).

I'VE READ THAT PROCESSED FOODS CAN CAUSE CANCER. IS THAT TRUE?

When meat is processed, preservatives are added (e.g., sodium nitrite or salt) to prevent the growth of bacteria, or the meat is smoked to preserve or enhance colors and flavors. These additives may include carcinogenic compounds. Several studies have shown that high consumption of processed meats is associated with an increased risk of colorectal and stomach cancer. This may be due to the nitrites frequently added to cold meats and cold cuts (deli meat, ham, and sausage) to preserve their color and prevent bacterial growth.[29]

MUST I AVOID PROCESSED MEATS?

Eating processed, smoked, or salt-cured meats increases your exposure to agents that may represent potential causes of cancer. That's why it is recommended to limit their consumption when possible.

DO IRRADIATED FOODS CAUSE CANCER?

Irradiation is widely used to preserve foods. It's one of the ways to limit the risk of germ contamination and food poisoning. Even though radiation is known to cause cancer, it does not remain in food after it's been irradiated, and consuming irradiated foods does not seem to affect or increase cancer risk. There is no evidence showing that irradiated foods cause cancer or have a harmful effect on human health.[30]

Resveratrol

DOES DRINKING A GLASS OF WINE DAILY REDUCE THE RISK OF CANCER?

Resveratrol is a natural antioxidant found in red and white wine, in the skin of grapes, blueberries, peanuts, pistachios, cacao, and dark chocolate. The plants these foods come from produce resveratrol to fight fungal infection and counteract the stress produced by ultraviolet radiation.

Due to their antioxidant and anti-inflammatory properties, resveratrol has received much attention from the media. Several studies suggest its possible use as an anticancer compound and protection against cardiovascular disease.[31] Furthermore, it could relieve the deleterious effects of anticancer treatments.

But studies on humans don't show the same results.[32] To get the anticancer benefits, we need to consume huge amounts of food rich in resveratrol. Resveratrol, due to its anti-inflammatory properties, might relieve cachexia (wasting away), lack of appetite, fatigue, weakness, and cognitive impairment frequently observed in people with advanced cancer. The same relief might also be obtained from regular exercise, good sleep, and anti-stress techniques (see chapter 5, "Energize Your Body!").

There are some precautions worth mentioning. Though it was proven that in some cases resveratrol may sensitize cells under chemotherapy, in other cases it might interfere in their mechanism and reduce the effectiveness of chemotherapy agents.[33] Other studies have also shown that since resveratrol is a phytoestrogen, it might activate genes that are normally regulated by estrogens and androgens. It would not be safe to recommend high doses of resveratrol for persons suffering from hormone-dependent cancer, for example breast cancer, uterine cancer, ovarian cancer, or prostate cancer.[34]

On the other hand, resveratrol makes platelets less "sticky" and enhances blood flow, but also increases the risk of bleeding in those taking anticoagulants such as warfarin, aspirin, and ibuprofen. Considering that the research on humans is not clear, taking resveratrol supplements is not recommended. You can ingest it in foods. If you decide to get your resveratrol in wine, women should consume only one glass per day and men not more than two.

Salt

DO LARGE AMOUNTS OF SALT INCREASE THE RISK OF CANCER?

There's much evidence that diets based on high amounts of salt-cured foods or foods prepared with vinegar have a higher risk of stomach cancer, nasopharyngeal cancer (a rare type of head and neck cancer), and throat cancer. A reduction in the consumption of salt-cured foods or foods prepared with vinegar might diminish the risk of these kinds of cancer.

Selenium

WHAT IS SELENIUM, AND HOW CAN IT REDUCE THE RISK OF CANCER?

Selenium is a mineral that boosts the body's immune system.[35] It might also reduce the immunologic hyperstimulation observed in some kinds of cancers such as leukemia, prostate cancer, and melanoma. The immune system is responsible for eliminating foreign substances from the body, including mutated cells—which are cancer precursors. Some kinds of cancer produce molecules that release in the blood and prevent the immune system from destroying cancer cells. Selenium neutralizes those substances and reestablishes the immune system's proper functioning.[36] The major food sources of selenium in the American diet are breads, grains, meat, poultry, fish, and eggs.[37]

Research studies in animals suggest that selenium might protect against some kinds of cancer. One study reported that selenium supplements might reduce the risk of lung, colon, and prostate cancer. But other studies couldn't prove it. Selenium supplements are therefore not recommended, and high doses of selenium supplements should be avoided, since there's a narrow margin between a safe dose and a toxic dose. If you choose to take a supplement for a limited time, the maximal dose should not exceed 200 micrograms per day.

Soy

NOW THAT I EAT LESS MEAT, I'VE STARTED EATING MORE TOFU AND

DRINKING SOY MILK. CAN MY BODY TAKE THIS MUCH SOY?

It's true that soy and tofu are alternatives to meat since they are good sources of protein. But there are two controversial factors: Soy contains phytoestrogens, and most soy sold today is genetically modified.

Phytoestrogens are chemical compounds, found in vegetables, that are similar to human estrogens and may have a similar effect. In regard to hormone-dependent cancer, like breast cancer, the research is not conclusive. Many studies show a reduction of the risk of breast cancer or its recurrence through taking soy products, but this this is not sufficiently conclusive to recommend supplementing diet with soy. For those whose diets already include soy products, there's evidence they can continue to do so safely. For those who do not eat soy products, the advice would be to continue avoiding soy, or if you incorporate soy into your diet, to do so only in moderate amounts.

GMO soybeans have been modified to tolerate herbicides, resist insects, and/or have better properties and nutrients. The long-term effects of consuming GMO soybeans are unknown (see "Genetically Modified Foods" in this glossary).

Sugar

CAN I CONSUME SUGAR, OR IS IT DANGEROUS? I WAS TOLD THAT CANCER FEEDS ON SUGAR.

In general, sugar is dangerous for health,[38] and according to many experts, it should be regulated similarly to tobacco and alcohol. An excess of sugar in food—refined or as sucrose or fructose additives—not only puts on weight, but also affects metabolism and brain function and makes us vulnerable to illness, such as cardiovascular disease, diabetes, and cancer. Besides, sugar is addictive. Eating it stimulates the same regions of the brain that are activated by alcohol and drugs. Sugar intake triggers the release of dopamine—the reward hormone, and of serotonin, which produces a soothing and therefore highly addictive effect.

It's recommended to drastically reduce sugar intake. Raising awareness and educating consumers is necessary but not sufficient, since most processed foods include some kind of sugar.

Whether sugar increases the risk of developing cancer and stimulating its growth is still under research and is a controversial issue.

Diabetics who have difficulty regulating blood sugar show an increase of different kinds of cancer,[39] but not all diabetic patients with an increased glycemic index develop cancer. Although a relation between diabetes and cancer has been observed, this does not mean sugar is the only cause. As of now, the mechanisms that link diabetes to some kinds of cancer are unknown.

Some interpreters of this data say cancer cells "feed on sugar," but actually all cells need sugar (glucose) as a source of energy. Increasing the level of sugar in the blood does not increase cancer cells' growth. This misunderstanding is based on the fact that glucose marked with a radioactive tracer is used to carry out a positron emission tomography (PET) scan, an X-ray study used in oncology that combines a CT scan with an analysis of how cells work. All cells absorb the marked glucose, but cells that are more active, such as cancer cells, absorb it to a higher extent. This is why it was concluded that cancer cells feed on glucose. But lab studies could not demonstrate that an increase of glycemia also increases the growth of cancer. So, it's possible that sugar is not responsible for this but reflects other imbalances, e.g. an increase of insulin[40] associated with other cell-growth factors[41] and obesity (most diabetic patients are obese or overweight). Sugar, and above all blood glucose peaks, may indirectly increase cancer risk and promote its development by increasing insulin levels in the body. That is why it's recommended to avoid blood glucose peaks by limiting the consumption of white flour (which rapidly breaks down into simple sugar), sweets, sugary drinks, adding sugar to coffee or tea, and even fruit and vegetable extracts (see "Juices" in this glossary). In some kinds of cancer, it's important to control *insulin levels* in blood rather than to control *sugar* in blood.

IF I STOP EATING SUGAR, WHAT ALTERNATIVE SWEETENERS ARE THERE? I'VE HEARD THAT OTHER SUGAR SUBSTITUTES CAUSE CANCER.

To date, there is no evidence that at the level of human consumption, artificial sweeteners such as aspartame, saccharin, and sucralose[42] cause cancer or increase the risk of developing cancer. However, it's advisable to stop consuming chemical additives in the diet (see "Additives" in this glossary). Stevia is a plant with sweetener properties that is recommended by many doctors and nutritionists as a replacement for sugar and artificial sweeteners.

Tea

DOES DRINKING GREEN OR BLACK TEA REDUCE THE RISK OF CANCER?

Tea is a beverage made by steeping leaves, buds, or twigs of the tea plant (*Camellia sinensis*) in hot water for a few minutes. Black, green, and white teas all derive from the same plant but are processed in different ways.

Research suggests that tea might have a protective effect against cancer due to its antioxidants, polyphenols, and flavonoids.

Green tea has anti-inflammatory and antioxidant properties and has been proven to have a protective effect against cancer. Green tea might enhance chemotherapy's anti-tumor effects and reduce its adverse effects.[43] But at times, it can reduce chemo's effectiveness (see e.g., green tea's interaction with bortezomib in "If it's sold over the counter, it's not a medicine and cannot interfere with my prescription drugs" under "Urban Legends" at the beginning of this appendix). The decision whether to drink green tea must be made with your doctor.

Though lab research studies show anticancer effects of black tea, research conducted on humans has not been conclusive.[44]

Turmeric

IS IT TRUE THAT TURMERIC REDUCES THE RISK OF CANCER?

Turmeric is a spice obtained from the aromatic rhizome of an Asian plant of the same name, cultivated mainly in India. **Curcumin** is a natural colorant deriving from turmeric, responsible for the color of *curry*. In addition to acting as an anti-inflammatory and having many other properties, curcumin is one of the most powerful regulators of the genes that cause cancer. Curcumin exerts its biological activities through epigenetic modulation. It changes the expression of DNA, activating genes that keep us healthy and deactivating ones that make us vulnerable to illness. Turmeric and its derivative curcumin reduce the risk of cancer.[45]

HOW CAN CURCUMIN BE USED?

Curcumin may be added, for example, to cooked vegetables, soups, or rice. It's important to take the recommended dosage and combine it with pepper to boost its absorption. Curry preparations often include curcumin and pepper, among other spices. It's advisable to prepare your own mix to be sure it includes your favorite ingredients.

Another way to enhance curcumin's absorption is by adding it to tea or preparing a curcumin infusion. Put one tablespoon of curcumin powder in a quart of boiling water. Boil for ten minutes. Allow it to cool, and drink throughout the day.[46]

SHOULD WE BE CAUTIOUS WHEN TAKING CURCUMIN?

Curcumin may have side effects in those suffering from gallstones or stomach ulcers or who have a propensity to kidney stones.

Curcumin interacts with many medicines. Recent research shows that it could inhibit the anticancer activity of chemotherapies cyclophosphamide and doxorubicin used to treat breast cancer.[47] Other medications curcumin could harmfully interact with are anticoagulants, some antibiotics, blood pressure medicines, and sleeping pills. On the other side, acetaminophen, aspirin, and ibuprofen may amplify curcumin's effects. Anyone undergoing chemotherapy or using other medications should ask their doctor about taking turmeric and determine the appropriate dosage.

Vitamins and Supplements

IS IT NECESSARY TO TAKE VITAMINS, MINERALS, OR OTHER SUPPLEMENTS?

In general, if you're consuming a diet rich in vegetables and fruits, and your digestive system functions normally, you are getting the required amounts of vitamins and minerals every day. But if your diet is deficient or you suffer digestive disorders or disorders in the absorption of food, or if you are under high stress, you might want to take supplements to ensure proper functioning.

WHICH SUPPLEMENTS MIGHT BE OF HELP? ON THE INTERNET I FOUND...[48]

As we saw at the beginning of this appendix (see "Natural products are better and aren't harmful" under "Urban Legends"), even supplements of natural origin are not always harmless. Supplements are marketed without rigorous research on what they contain, what their adverse effects might be, or how they interact with other medications.

Some supplements do not contain what is written on the label; some are contaminated; some have filler substances that may have undesirable effects and aren't on the label; some have compounds or medications added to give them additional properties, e.g., amphetamines added to herbs used to lose weight. To avoid taking supplements that might have side effects, it's best to avoid products that say they produce the effects of a medication or promise miracle cures.

There's information on the internet that guarantees a cure for cancer with supplements. In general, these have no scientific or solid basis. The research studies on nutritional supplements to reduce the risk of cancer have not been disappointing, but most do not support their use for the purpose of reducing the risk of cancer.

A diet rich in fruits, vegetables, and grains helps reduce the risk of cancer, but there's not much evidence that nutritional supplements have the same effect. Food already has vitamins, minerals, and other substances that have beneficial effects for health due to their complex interactions with each other. In an orange, we will find vitamin C, but eating an orange is not the same as taking a supplement that only contains that vitamin. In the orange, vitamin C is combined with other vitamins and minerals, and its beneficial effects may be enhanced from this combination. The best advice is to **eat whole foods as part of a balanced diet.**

Most of the proposed supplements with anticancer effects act on animals, but not on humans. Every year, tests are conducted on a large number of compounds to analyze their effects on the reduction of tumors. Among the few compounds that show anticancer activity on animals, fewer than 5 percent are effective on humans.[49] Why then are supplements to reduce cancer so widely promoted? The nutritional supplements business is huge. In the US, it's more than $20 billion per year. The approval process of a nutritional supplement is much less rigorous than that of a drug. Thus, many manufacturers try to sell substances with therapeutic purposes under the guise of nutritional supplements. Among these, we can find real nutritional supplements and other compounds that claim to have multiple therapeutic benefits that are not yet proven.[50]

General advice is to focus on a healthy diet. We can supplement our diet **for a limited time by adding balanced multivitamin and mineral supplements** with a content lower than the recommended 100 percent daily dose.[51]

For all remaining supplements, it's wise to proceed with caution and always make decisions based on real information, particularly if you're undergoing chemotherapy, since other substances could counteract chemo's effectiveness. And during periods without treatment, it's advisable to avoid the use of supplements that might have side effects unless you are certain the supplements will be beneficial for you.

Each person must decide, with the aid of a doctor, if supplements should be taken, and if so, which are the most appropriate for the situation. Priority should be given to those with scientific evidence affirming their usefulness and safety, and to avoid those that haven't been sufficiently tested. The decision whether to take supplements will change according to your needs and the results of tests in progress.

VITAMIN A AND CAROTENE

Does vitamin A reduce the risk of cancer?

Vitamin A (retinol) is necessary to keep tissue healthy. It can be obtained from foods of animal origin or by beta-carotene or other carotenoids in foods of plant origin.

Vitamin A supplements have not been proven to reduce the risk of cancer, and supplements containing high doses of vitamin A may actually increase the risk of developing lung cancer in smokers and ex-smokers.

Does beta-carotene reduce the risk of cancer?

Beta-carotene belongs to a group of antioxidants known as carotenoids and is the source of the intense orange color of many plants, including fruits and vegetables. In the body, beta-carotene is transformed into vitamin A. Since the consumption of fruits and vegetables has been associated with a reduction in the risk of cancer, it would be reasonable to think that taking beta-carotene supplements would produce the same result. However, large-scale research studies have not proven it.[52] Consuming fruits and vegetables that contain beta-carotene may be beneficial, but high doses of beta-carotene supplements should be avoided.

VITAMIN B: FOLATE, FOLIC ACID, AND NIACIN

What is folate and folic acid, and can they reduce the risk of cancer?

Folate and folic acid are part of the vitamin B complex naturally found in many vegetables, such as spinach and lettuce; beans and chickpeas; whole grains and fortified cereals. Since it is heat- and light-sensitive, it is better found in raw food.

Folate and folic acid protect the DNA of chromosomes in the event of viral injuries. Research studies suggest that lack of folate could increase the risk of colorectal, liver, uterine, cervical, and breast cancer. The best way to ingest folate is by eating fruits, vegetables, and products with whole or enriched grains. Meat is low in folic acid. If an unhealthy diet lacks folic acid, compounded by being meat-based, it can be helpful to consume processed foods enriched with folates.

Niacin, a B vitamin (B3), is also necessary for our health. It's a strong cell-degeneration inhibitor and acts in the metabolism of carbohydrates, fats, and proteins. You can get niacin by eating whole grains, avocados, figs, and plums.

VITAMIN C

Does vitamin C reduce the risk of cancer?

Vitamin C is found in many fruits and vegetables, particularly oranges, grapefruits, and peppers. Several studies have found a relation between consuming foods rich in vitamin C and lowering the risk of cancer. However, the few studies in which *supplements* have been the source of vitamin C did not show a reduction in the risk of cancer. (See appendix 2, "Frequently Asked Questions About Treatment.")

VITAMIN D

Do I have to take vitamin D supplements?

Vitamin D helps metabolize calcium. Studies have shown that vitamin D protects against cancer.[53]

Skin exposed to the sun's rays may produce vitamin D. You can also find it in certain foods, such as fatty fish, fish liver, and egg yolks. Many dairy products are fortified with vitamin D.

Ultraviolet sun rays activate the pro-vitamin D in the skin and transform it into vitamin D, which is subsequently activated by the liver and kidney to be usable. It's important to monitor your levels of vitamin D every six months, since they change from person to person depending on ultraviolet exposure and diet. To optimize your health, your serum level (25, OH cholecalciferol, the active form) should be between 50 and 70 nanograms per milliliter (ng/ml). When values are lower, you can take vitamin supplements to normalize these levels. The US National Academies of Sciences, Engineering and Medicine, Health and Medicine Division, recently increased the recommended daily consumption of vitamin D based on the levels required for bone health, from 400 to 600 international units per day for most adults, and 800 international units for those over the age of seventy. The upper daily limit considered safe was increased from 2,000 to 4,000 international units.

VITAMIN E

Does vitamin E reduce the risk of cancer?

Alpha-Tocopherol, a powerful antioxidant, is the most active form of vitamin E in humans. Research studying its efficacy preventing cancer has had mixed results. One study showed that smokers taking alpha-Tocopherol had a lower risk of prostate cancer than those who took only a placebo. This resulted in a large-scale study, known as SELECT,[54] that analyzed the effects of selenium and vitamin E supplements on prostate cancer. This survey reported that they didn't reduce the risk of prostate cancer. In fact, men who took the vitamin E supplement might have increased their risk. Another large-scale survey, known as HOPE,[55] analyzed the risk of cancer and heart disease when taking vitamin E supplements compared with a placebo, and there was no difference between the groups.

Vitamin E *supplements* are not recommended for reducing the risk of cancer or chronic diseases, though many foods that contain vitamin E, including nuts and some unsaturated oils, have shown a reduction of the risk of heart disorders.

VITAMIN K2

A friend told me about vitamin K. What do you know about it in relation to cancer?

Lab research studies with animals suggest that vitamin K2 might have protective effects against prostate cancer.[56] Tests on humans are still in progress.

Vitamin K is a fat-soluble vitamin and can be obtained from fatty foods, such as raw cheese. There are also supplements.

Vitamin K is an antidote for anticoagulants, so its use in supplements is not recommended for anyone undergoing anticoagulation treatments or suffering from cardio- or cerebrovascular diseases or thrombosis.

Weight

DOES BEING OVERWEIGHT INCREASE THE RISK OF CANCER?

There is clear evidence that being overweight, and especially being obese, increases the risk of esophageal, kidney, pancreatic, colon, rectal, breast (in women after menopause), and endometrial cancer, and it predisposes people to an increase of the risk of gallbladder, liver, non-Hodgkin lymphoma, multiple myeloma, uterine, cervical, ovarian, and aggressive forms of prostate cancer.

It's important for overweight people to try to lose weight and stay fit. This reduces the risk of cancer and other chronic diseases.[57]

WHAT IS MY HEALTHIEST WEIGHT?

To determine the healthiest weight for a person, body mass index (BMI) is used. BMI is calculated using your height and weight. There are apps for calculating these values, or just go to google.com and type in "BMI."

In general, the higher the value, the larger amount of body fat you have, although it can differ between women and men. A high BMI shows a higher risk of developing heart diseases, diabetes, and cancer.

For most adults, a healthy BMI ratio is between 18.5 and 25. A BMI between 25 and 30 means you're overweight, and a BMI higher than 30 represents obesity.

WHAT IS THE BEST WAY TO LOSE WEIGHT?

Losing weight doesn't mean giving up eating. The best way to achieve a healthy body weight is by balancing energy consumed (what we eat and drink) with energy expended (physical activity). The excess of body fat may be reduced by decreasing the number of calories consumed *and* increasing physical activity.

Eat and drink the quantities necessary to help you achieve and maintain a healthy weight.

1. Read the nutritional labels on foods to be more aware of the number of calories and size of portions. Bear in mind that

"low-fat" and "nonfat" do not necessarily mean "low-calorie."

2. Eat smaller portions of high-calorie food.

3. Choose fruits, vegetables, and other foods low in calories, instead of foods with high calorie content, like potato chips, ice cream, pastries, and sweets.

4. Eat a variety of vegetables every day, at least 2 1/2 cups (or 5 units). Include fruits and vegetables with each meal and for snacks. If you drink juices, be sure they're 100 percent pure, without added sugars or taste enhancers.

5. Reduce quantities of creamy sauces, dressings, and dips on fruits and vegetables.

6. Reduce consumption of sugar-sweetened beverages, e.g., soft drinks, energy drinks, and beverages with artificial fruit flavors.

7. When you eat in restaurants, be careful to choose foods with low-calorie contents—less fat and

added sugar—and avoid large portions.

Zinc

DO I HAVE TO TAKE ZINC?
Low levels of zinc have been associated with an increase of cancer. Zinc strengthens the immune system, and its levels should be kept in healthy ranges to stay healthy. Small doses of zinc can be found in shellfish, legumes, Brewer's yeast, wheat germ, eggs, and milk.[58]

Reference Sites

For more information, see:

American Cancer Society, "ACS Guidelines on Nutrition and Physical Activity for Cancer Prevention." www.cancer.org/healthy/eat-healthy-get-active/acs-guidelines-nutrition-physical-activity-cancer-prevention.html

Memorial Sloan Kettering Cancer Center, "About Herbs, Botanicals & Other Products." www.mskcc.org/cancer-care

/diagnosis-treatment/symptom-manage
ment/integrative-medicine/herbs

Dr. Odile Fernández is a medical doctor
who survived cancer. She offers her
recommendations at www.misrecetasan
ticancer.com (in Spanish).

Shopping List

This list can be helpful as a
guideline for buying healthy foods.

Vegetables and legumes

- artichoke
- arugula
- asparagus
- avocado
- beets
- broccoli
- Brussels sprouts
- cauliflower
- celery
- chicory
- chives
- collard greens or kale
- cucumber
- dandelion leaves

- endive
- escarole
- fennel
- garlic
- green onion
- green or red cabbage
- leeks
- Napa cabbage, Chinese cabbage, or bok choy
- onion
- parsley
- pepper: red, green, yellow, and hot
- romaine lettuce, red lettuce, green lettuce
- rutabaga
- spinach
- Swiss chard
- tomato
- turnip
- zucchini

Eggplants, winter squash, jicama, beets, and carrots should be consumed moderately due to their high levels of carbohydrates.

Mushrooms

- Japanese mushrooms, such as shiitake or maitake

Fruits

- black grapes
- citrus fruits, particularly lemon
- pineapple
- red fruits, especially blueberries
- umeboshi plums, common in Japanese cuisine

Seeds

- flaxseeds

Cereals

- oats

Spices and dressings

- ginger
- olive oil
- turmeric

Miscellaneous

- green tea
- red wine
- water kefir

Appendix 2

FREQUENTLY ASKED QUESTIONS ABOUT TREATMENT

Can I take vitamins, supplements, or herbs during treatment?

As we saw in the "Vitamins and Supplements" entry in the glossary in appendix 1, a well-balanced diet generally offers the vitamins and minerals the body needs for daily activities. Sometimes during treatment, however, due to lack of appetite or gastrointestinal disorders, it is necessary to take supplements to be sure the daily recommended doses of vitamins and minerals are met.

If you choose to take supplements, especially during an anticancer treatment, it's advisable to analyze the pros and cons of each with a doctor or a nutritionist, since many supplements can cause adverse interactions with chemo and/or radiation.

- Some dietary supplements may cause skin hypersensitivity and severe reactions if taken during radiation.
- Some vitamins may interact with chemo or radiation in a way that increases their adverse effects or reduces their effectiveness. That's why high doses of vitamins are not recommended during treatment.
- Many medicinal plants and supplements alter the healing mechanisms and interfere with certain anesthetics. If you have a surgery or invasive test scheduled, you should suspend treatments with natural plants and supplements for twelve to fifteen days prior.
- Anticoagulants (heparin, warfarin, acenocoumarol) or antiplatelet drugs (aspirin, dipyridamole) are commonly used in oncology to prevent or treat complications of treatment or the disease. These are known for their interaction with other medications, but also with herbs and supplements. Anyone

undergoing anticoagulant treatments must see an integrative doctor beforehand to determine which supplements they can or cannot take.

- Studies on selenium supplements show mixed results. Some surveys on patients receiving chemo showed a better response to treatment with selenium, but another survey on the prevention of prostate cancer showed no benefit at all. Many kinds of cancer, for example melanoma, prostate cancer, and some leukemias, produce an overstimulation of the immune system leading it to fail. It appears that selenium might reduce the immune response and enhance the cancer treatment.[1] The accumulation of selenium in the body is toxic, which is why advice whether or not to take selenium supplements must be tailored for each person.

- Though zinc deficiency prevents the proper functioning of the immune system, an excess of zinc inhibits it. This is why zinc supplements are recommended only in cases of deficiency.

Is orthomolecular medicine useful?

Micronutrients are substances we need in small doses, such as iodine, selenium, and vitamin A, for the proper functioning of our metabolism and body in general. Orthomolecular medicine is based on the hypothesis that if the body receives the necessary micronutrients, many diseases can be prevented, and if the disease is already present, it can be partially or totally cured.

The application of orthomolecular medicine in oncology is based on the scientific observations of Linus Pauling on vitamin C, which could not be confirmed (see chapter 2, "So ... What Is Cancer?"). Today orthomolecular medicine usually refers to a therapy based mainly on megadoses of vitamins (e.g., vitamin C), minerals, or hormones—considerably higher than daily recommended doses. This medicine is also known as megavitamin and mega-mineral therapy or nutritional medicine.

It's true that when the disease occurs, the person's diet might be inadequate and vitamin and mineral supplements might be necessary to correct deficiencies. For example, after a long period of high stress, not only is our ability to digest food properly reduced (because stress produces substances that impair digestion), but fast food diets we resort to when we have little time available are of a low quality. Since the body must function properly to eliminate these substances, taking supplements can be advisable, though not necessarily in megadoses. This is because many supplements are antioxidants, which counteract the effect of free radicals produced during stress.

Cancer-prevention studies show that the intake of supplements is less effective than eating fruits and vegetables, which are already rich in vitamins and minerals. There are other beneficial substances in fruits and vegetables, and the combinations of vitamins and minerals in fruits and vegetables may make them more effective than supplements.

On some occasions, high doses of vitamins and minerals may be harmful. For example, the accumulation of vitamins A and D, or of minerals such as selenium, iron, magnesium, zinc, and other compounds, may cause certain disorders. An overdose of minerals may cause vomiting, diarrhea, hair loss, and changes in skin and nails. High doses of vitamin A may produce headaches, dizziness, irritability, vomiting, and changes in skin and nails. Overdoses of vitamin D may reduce appetite and cause nausea, vomiting, weakness, and kidney disorders. In some cases, the intake of supplements increases the risk of cancer.

In a 1996 research study, people with a high risk of developing cancer because they smoked or had been exposed to asbestos were treated with vitamin A with the intent of reducing the risk. Researchers found out that the group receiving vitamins was more likely to develop lung cancer and cardiovascular disease, and their mortality rate was higher. The study was immediately stopped, but researchers continued to monitor the people in the study and observed that while the cardiovascular disease risk was reduced over time, cancer risk levels remained high for many years.[2] Another study was designed to evaluate the effects of vitamins A and E in reducing the adverse effects of radiation therapy. Even though those taking vitamins showed fewer adverse effects, they also had more recurrences of their cancer. This suggests that the antioxidants taken during treatment reduced the treatment's effectiveness.[3]

Scientific studies do not support the use of orthomolecular therapy, especially in high doses, for most of the diseases it's being used for. There's no evidence that vitamin or mineral supplements, by themselves, cure cancer.

Is it true that homeopathy may help?

Homeopathy is a system of alternative medicine created in 1796 by Samuel Hahnemann, based on the doctrine of "like cures like," that a substance that causes the symptoms of a disease in healthy people would cure similar symptoms in sick people. Homeopathy is well respected and used in several countries. It is not unanimously accepted by science, because while some clinical studies in cancer patients have shown favorable results, others have not.[4] Many of these studies, however, were not adequately designed to evaluate it. These treatments cannot be studied by analyzing large populations and average results, because homeopathic treatments are personalized, and averaging conclusions cannot show each person's unique and significant differences. Since homeopathy is focused on a holistic perspective, it's also not relevant to analyze isolated symptoms in a reductionist manner, without considering its role affecting the person as a whole.

Homeopathy helps certain people stimulate their immune systems, tolerate treatments better, and improve the quality of their life. Each person needs to decide with his or her reliable homeopath if there is an adequate treatment available.

Is it true that eating mushrooms can help?

There are many different kinds of mushrooms. Shiitake and maitake mushrooms from Asia are among the best known. It's been shown that these mushrooms are beneficial for the organism.[5]

Shiitake in particular has brought about improvements in the quality of life of patients with liver, stomach, colon, and pancreatic cancer.[6] These mushrooms can also reduce adverse effects of chemotherapy.[7] Although scientific studies to determine the benefits of mushrooms during chemo are still being conducted, adding mushrooms to the diet is a good idea.

Maitake mushrooms are sold as supplements to "stimulate the immune system." Although some preliminary studies show favorable results,[8] diabetic patients, those taking hypoglycemic medications, and those undergoing anticoagulant treatment need to consult their physicians before consuming maitake mushrooms because they interfere with these medications and can produce severe side effects.[9]

Is graviola (soursop) recommended?

Graviola is a fruit tree that grows in tropical regions. Extracts from different parts of the graviola fruit have shown anticancer properties in lab studies on animals but have not yet been proven on humans.

Some substances deriving from graviola species harm nervous cells and may cause symptoms similar to Parkinson's disease. They may also cause toxicity in the liver and kidneys and interfere with sensitivity to radiological studies.

Due to the lack of proven effectiveness and the possibility of neurological harm, graviola cannot be recommended.[10]

So-Called "Anticancer" Products

Several over-the-counter products are promoted as "anticancer" based on studies with animals. It's estimated that 95 percent of the compounds that reduce tumors in animals are not effective for humans.[11]

Studies conducted on animals provide useful guidelines but cannot be considered evidence of effectiveness in people.

What about Viscum?

Viscum album is one of 100 species of mistletoe. Preparations made from European mistletoe (Viscum album, Loranthaceae) are among the most prescribed drugs offered to cancer patients.

Mistletoe and its derivatives have proven to stimulate components of the immune system and have anticancer activity in the lab. Some studies with Viscum on humans have shown positive results, while others have had negative results. Preliminary studies in humans show the efficiency of Viscum to improve symptoms and reduce the effects of chemo and/or radiation.

Viscum is used to improve the adverse effects of chemotherapy and the quality of life. For patients under gemcitabine chemotherapy, Viscum allowed for higher gemcitabine doses without major toxicity. It cannot be considered an agent useful to prevent or treat cancer. Before using Viscum, all possible interactions with other medications must be taken into account.[12]

Where can we find more information?

More information about cancer can be found at the following sites:

- American Cancer Society: www.cancer.org
- Society of Integrative Oncology: https://integrativeonc.org

For more information on nutrition, visit:

- Academy of Nutrition and Dietetics: www.oncologynutrition.org/erfc/eating-well-when-unwell/white-blood-count-diet
- Odile Fernández's website: www.misrecetasanticancer.com

For more information on how to deal with cancer, visit:

- Cancer Care: www.cancercare.org
  To know more about herbs and phytotherapy, consult:
- Memorial Sloan Kettering Cancer Center: www.mskcc.org/cancer-care/diagnosis-treatment/symptom-management/integrative-medicine/herbs

This site includes updated information from specialized scientists and researchers. The site uses technical language for professionals as well as general language for the public.

Appendix 3

THE CHAKRA SYSTEM[1]

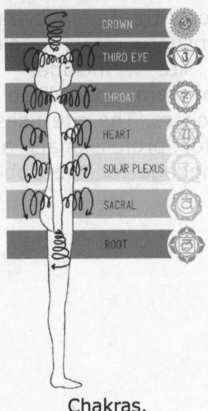

Chakras.

1. Root Chakra

This first chakra is located at the base of the spine. Its main color is **red,** and it vibrates at the frequency of the **musical note C.** One might say that we are spirits embodied in order to have a human experience. With that image in mind, this chakra is essential for an earthly life because it's related to being **grounded** and connected with the earth's biological cycles and meeting the basic needs of food, clothing, and shelter. Our **legs** are an extension of this chakra. They are our roots.

The main function of the root chakra is related to physical survival. In ancient times, survival required being in contact with the earth, going out hunting or gathering, and eventually cultivating. Nowadays, survival is associated with having enough money to meet our basic needs. When this chakra is balanced, we're able to survive without effort, either by earning our own money or cultivating our own food.

This chakra can be knocked off balance by the fear of not being able to provide for basic needs, which today means not having enough money. When this chakra is out of balance, we're ungrounded, don't feel anchored to everyday life, fail to develop normally, don't enjoy our work, and our work doesn't meet our needs.

2. Sacral Chakra

The second chakra is located above the pubic bone and below the navel. It vibrates with the color **orange** and the sound of the **musical note D.** This chakra distributes energy to the **kidneys** and **reproductive organs.** It regulates sexuality, the **possibility of creating and procreating, and achieving creativity and pleasure.**

When this chakra is balanced, we're creative in everyday life, able to find solutions to problems, find sexuality really pleasant, and may get involved in artistic activities.

The emotion that blocks this chakra is **guilt.** When it's out of balance, we may feel a blockage in creativity and will not enjoy our sexuality.

3. Solar Plexus Chakra

The solar plexus is located in the **pit of the stomach.** This third chakra vibrates with the color **yellow** and the sound of the **musical note E.** It is our sun. It regulates the energy of the

digestive system, including the pancreas.

Through the third chakra, **we relate to other people,** position ourselves in the world, and fortify our place in it. The third chakra is associated with self, personality, and ego. It is the place where self-esteem and willpower reside.

When our third chakra is balanced, we feel self-confident and empowered.

Shame brings the third chakra out of balance. We're concerned about what others think and what society expects of us, and we become insecure and suffer from low self-esteem. Some people, when not in balance, might feel inflated, or high self-esteem. Still others might be indecisive or find it hard to set limits or say no. Some may feel anger, alienation, or loss.

In general in the West, our third chakras are out of balance, as we normally identify ourselves with our achievements, profession, material status, and being accepted by others, rather than with who we really are.

4. Heart Chakra

The fourth chakra is located in the center of the **chest** and extends to the arms and hands. This chakra vibrates with the color **green** and the sound of the **musical note F.**

We can connect with its energy in the center of the chest. This chakra regulates the **heart, lungs, thymus gland, and breasts** in both women and men.

The fourth chakra regulates our **ability to love;** it balances our ability to give and receive love. As a part of our heart chakra, the breasts hold our capacity to love as well as our deepest emotional wounds.

A person with a balanced and open fourth chakra is loving, with confidence in life and feelings of well-being, joy, and compassion.

When this chakra is out of balance, we become **suspicious, unhappy, and depressed.** Often when we don't accept a pain that has arisen from life, we begin to suffer, and our heart chakra becomes closed and imbalanced.

The heart chakra is the gateway to evolution and growth. It's the wellspring of love and the key to healing.

5. Throat Chakra

The fifth chakra is associated with communication. It is located in the **throat** and vibrates with the color **turquoise** and the sound of **the musical note G.** This chakra nourishes the **thyroid gland** by balancing its energy. It also radiates energy to the **tongue, vocal cords,** and **mouth.**

Someone who has an open throat chakra can **express his or her feelings clearly and is honest with him- or herself.**

When this chakra is out of balance, communication problems arise. We're unable or afraid to say what we want to say or express our feelings in a way that damages a connection with someone we value. This chakra gets out of balance for lack of honesty or hiding feelings.

6. Third-Eye

This is the **intuition** chakra and is related to our ability to see beyond space and time. It is known as the **third eye,** located **in the middle of our forehead.** This chakra vibrates with the color **indigo, or violet,** and with the sound of the **musical note A.**

It radiates vital energy to the **pituitary gland,** involved in regulating the entire hormonal system. It also radiates energy to the eyes, ears, and face. The third-eye chakra is our **guiding star.**

Those within whom this chakra is open and balanced enjoy **intuition, wisdom, and imagination.** They are able to understand the meaning of dreams, interpret experiences with a wide view, and give a deeper meaning to life's experiences.

When this chakra is out of balance, we feel lost in space and time and lack discernment. We feel as though we're **trapped in an illusion,** unable to see the truth behind the veils. When we feel this way, it's easy for others to lure us and to get us to believe ideologies or marketing campaigns.

7. Crown Chakra

The crown chakra, located at the **top of the head** as its name suggests, is the gateway to higher dimensions, the "kingdom of heaven." It's associated with **violet or white light** and vibrates to the sound of the **musical note B.**

The crown chakra radiates vital energy to the **pineal gland,** involved in the regulation of the sleep–wake cycle, daydreaming, and the regulation of the PNIE system. Many people see this chakra light easily, and artists portray a subject who has this chakra open, for example saints, with a white or golden aura (halo) around their head. Those within whom this chakra is balanced are able to experience union with all beings in the universe. People for whom this chakra is out of balance or closed live a **purely earthly life.**

NOTES

Acknowledgments

[1]   Inspired by "Gracias a la Vida," thanks to life, the name of a well-known Chilean folk song by Violeta Parra.

Chapter 1

[1]   V. RajMohan and E. Mohandas, "The Limbic System," *Indian Journal of Psychiatry* 49, no 2 (April–June 2007): 132–139. www.indianjpsychiatry.org/article.asp?issn=0019-5545;year=2007;volume=49;issue=2;spage=132;epage=139;aulast=RajMohan

[2]   The definition is in the Preamble to the Constitution of the World Health Organization as adopted by the International Health Conference, New York, June 19–22, 1946; signed on July 22, 1946, by the representatives of 61 States (*Official Records of the World Health Organization,* no.2, 100) and entered into force on

April 7, 1948. The definition has not been amended since 1948. See www.who.int/suggestions/faq/en/

[3] Many reports show that patients request to be treated as a whole person, paying attention to all their physical, emotional, family, and spiritual needs. One of these is Tracy A. Balboni et al., "Religiousness and Spiritual Support Among Advanced Cancer Patients and Associations with End-of-Life Treatment Preferences and Quality of Life," *Journal of Clinical Oncology* 25, no.5 (2007): 555–560. doi:10.1200/JCO.2006.07.9046

[4] National Cancer Institute, "Harms of Cigarette Smoking and Health Benefits of Quitting." www.cancer.gov/about-cancer/causes-prevention/risk/tobacco/cessation-fact-sheet

[5] Mary Ann Sens et al., "Unexpected Neoplasia in Autopsies: Potential Implications for Tissue and Organ Safety," *Archives of Pathology &*

Laboratory Medicine 133, no.12 (December 2009): 1923–1931.

[6] Sante Basso Ricci and Ugo Cerchiari, "Spontaneous Regression of Malignant Tumors: Importance of the Immune System and Other Factors (review)," *Oncology Letters* 1, no.6 (2010): 941–945. doi:10.3 892/ol.2010.176

[7] American Cancer Society, "Cancer Facts & Figures 2016." www.can cer.org/content/dam/cancer-org/ research/cancer-facts-and-statist ics/annual-cancer-facts-and-figur es/2016/cancer-facts-and-figures -2016.pdf

[8] World Health Organization, "Cancer Fact Sheet February 2017." www.who.int/mediacentre /factsheets/fs297

[9] WHO, "Cancer Fact Sheet."

[10] ACS, "Cancer Facts & Figures."

Chapter 2

[1] Laura J. Esserman, Ian M. Thompson Jr, and Brian Reid, "Overdiagnosis and

Overtreatment in Cancer: An Opportunity for Improvement," *Journal of the American Medical Association* 310, no.8 (2013): 797–798.

[2]   Rose Eveleth, "There are 37.2 Trillion Cells in Your Body," Smithsonian.com (October 24, 2013). www.smithsonianmag.com/smart-news/there-are-372-trillion-cells-in-your-body-4941473/

[3]   Deoxyribonucleic acid is the raw material of a gene. A gene is a sequence of nucleotides within the molecule of DNA that contains the information necessary to synthesize a macromolecule with specific cell function, normally a protein.

[4]   Bruce Lipton, *The Biology of Belief: Unleashing the Power of Consciousness* (Carlsbad, Calif.: Hay House, 2008), 37–42.

[5]   In Hans Selye's book, *The Stress of Life* (New York: McGraw-Hill, 1976), which was first published in his native Hungary in 1964, he introduced the term *stressors* to refer to the causes of stress,

such as hatred, anxiety, fear, frustration, noise, and nicotine.

[6]   Boudewijn J.M. Braakhuis et al., "A Genetic Explanation of Slaughter's Concept of Field Cancerization Evidence and Clinical Implications 1," *Cancer Research* 63, no.8 (April 15, 2003): 1727–1730. http://cancerres.aacrjournals.org/content/canres/63/8/1727.full.pdf

[7]   Natalie Ja□ger et al., "Hypermutation of the Inactive X Chromosome Is a Frequent Event in Cancer," *Cell* 155, no.3 (Oct 24, 2013): 567–581. doi:10.1016/j.cell.2013.09.042

[8]   John Cairns, Julie Overbaugh, and Stephan Miller, "The Origin of Mutants," *Nature* (London) 335 (1988): 142–145. www.ncbi.nlm.nih.gov/pubmed/3045565

[9]   Chemical process in which oxygen is used to produce energy as from carbohydrates (sugars). Also called aerobic metabolism, aerobic respiration, or cellular respiration.

[10]   Otto Warburg professed that cancer could be cured if one could identify metabolic differences between cancer cells and normal cells. His studies were carried out in histological preparations, and he could never show that the oxygen used by normal and cancer cells is different. He did find that cancer cells produced lactate in the presence of oxygen and glucose, while normal cells produced lactate in the absence of oxygen. This observation led him to conclude that the mechanisms to produce energy in the cells were defective in cancer cells and that this difference could be used to design treatments to favor normal energy-producing mechanisms that would make the normal cells outgrow the cancerous ones. Otto A. Warburg, "A Review," *Science* I 23 (1956): 309–315.

[11] Alan Clifford Aisenberg, *The Glycolysis and Respiration of Tumors. A Review* (New York: Academic Press, 1961).

[12] Edward T. Creagan, Charles G. Moertel, Judith R. O'Fallon, Allan J. Schutt, Michael J. O'Connell, Joseph Rubin, and Stephen Frytak, "Failure of High-Dose Vitamin C (Ascorbic Acid) Therapy to Benefit Patients with Advanced Cancer. A Controlled Trial," *New England Journal of Medicine* 301, no.13 (September 27, 1979): 687–690. doi:10.1056/NEJM197909273011303

[13] Wilhelm Reich, *The Cancer Biopathy: The Discovery of Orgone,* Vol.2 (New York: Farrar, Straus and Giroux, 1974).

[14] Steven A. Roberts and Dmitry A. Gordenin, "Hypermutation in Human Cancer Genomes: Footprints and Mechanisms," *Nature Reviews Cancer* 14, no.12 (2014): 786–800. doi 10.1038/nrc3816 and Evan

Harris Walker, "Cancer as a Mechanism of Hypermutation," *Acta Biotheoretica* 40, no.1 (March 1992): 31–40.

[15] Longchenpa, *Now That I Come to Die* (Cazadero, Calif.: Dharma Publishing, 2007).

[16] Hisae Iinuma et al., "Clinical Significance of Circulating Tumor Cells, Including Cancer Stem-Like Cells, in Peripheral Blood for Recurrence and Prognosis in Patients with Dukes' Stage B and C Colorectal Cancer," *Journal of Clinical Oncology* 29, no.12 (April 20, 2011): 1547–1555.

[17] Renee L. Manser et al., "Incidental Lung Cancers Identified at Coronial Autopsy: Implications for Overdiagnosis of Lung Cancer by Screening," *Respiratory Medicine* 99, no.4 (2005): 501–507. www.resmed journal.com/article/S0954-6111 (04)00335-X/pdf and S.G. Silverberg. "The Autopsy and Cancer," *Archives of Pathology*

& *Laboratory Medicine* 108, no.6 (June 1984): 476–478.

[18] Per-Henrik Zahl, Jan Mæhlen, and H. Gilbert Welch, "The Natural History of Breast Cancers Detected by Screening Mammography," *Archives of Pathology & Laboratory Medicine* 168, no.231 (2008): 1–6, and Per-Henrik Zahl, Peter C. Gøtzsche, and Jan Mæhlen, "Natural History of Breast Cancer Detected in the Swedish Mammography Screening Programme: A Cohort Study," *Lancet Oncology* 12, no.11 (November 12, 2011): 18–24.

[19] Michael Gnant et al., "Endocrine Therapy plus Zoledronic Acid in Premenopausal Breast Cancer," *New England Journal of Medicine* 360 (February 12, 2009): 679–691. doi:10.1056/NEJMoa0806285

[20] Psycho-neuro-immuno-endocrinology (PNIE) is a term coined by Robert Ader and Nicholas Cohen in 1991 to define the communication and

inter-modulation between psychical processes, the nervous system, the immune system, and the endocrine system. It's an interdisciplinary field of study, and receives contributions from psychology, psychiatry, neuroscience, pharmacology, molecular science, endocrinology, and i m m u n o l o g y . Psycho-neuro-immuno-endocrinology gives a scientific basis for how psychosocial factors affect immune and hormonal responses, e.g., how chronic stress depresses the immune system and is thus responsible for some diseases.

[21] See chapter 7, "The Treasure Hunt."

Chapter 3

[1] Stents are mesh devices inserted in the lumen of a vessel (a coronary artery, or any artery or vein) to help keep a blocked passageway open.

[2]   The World Health Organization described labor stress as epidemic. A United Nations report issued in the 1990s labeled job stress "the 20th century disease."

[3]   Instead of evaluating stress directly, it's more effective to evaluate its symptoms, such as anxiety, hostility, and depression. See Selye, *The Stress of Life.*

[4]   H.W.L. Poonja, *This: Prose and Poetry of Dancing Emptiness* (Newburyport, Mass.: Red Wheel/Weiser, 2000), 69.

[5]   J. Bruce Moseley et al., "A Controlled Trial of Arthroscopic Surgery for Osteoarthritis of the Knee," *New England Journal of Medicine* 347, no.2 (July 11, 2002): 81–88.

[6]   For an excellent explanation of how the placebo effect works, see Joe Dispenza, *You Are the Placebo: Making Your Mind Matter* (Carlsbad, Calif.: Hay House, 2015).

[7]   For an excellent description of how fear can either make us sick

or enlighten us, see Lissa Rankin, *The Fear Cure: Cultivating Courage as Medicine for the Body, Mind, and Soul* (Carlsbad, Calif.: Hay House, 2016).

[8] This story is told in Paul Reps, *Zen Flesh, Zen Bones: A Collection of Zen and Pre-Zen Writings* (Rutland, VT: Tuttle Publishing, 1998), 39.

[9] Julie Cahu, "SASP: Roadblock for Tissue Reorganization," *Aging* 5, no.9 (2013): 641–642. www.im pactaging.com/papers/v5/n9/full/ 100602.html

[10] Luc Besson created the film *Lucy* (2014) based on this concept.

[11] See Fritjof Capra and Pier Luigi Luisi, *The Systems View of Life: A Unifying Vision* (New York: Cambridge University Press, 2016).

[12] Danny Hillis, "Understanding Cancer Through Proteomics," TEDMED 2010. www.ted.com/t alks/danny_hillis_two_frontiers_ of_cancer_treatment

Chapter 4

[1]   Wayne Muller, *A Life of Being, Having, and Doing Enough* (New York: Harmony Books, 2011), 98.

[2]   Francisco Varela, Humberto Maturana, Ilya Prigogine, Edgar Morin, and others call this the *complexity paradigm.*

[3]   More about the factors that, in isolation or in combination, may cause an imbalance in the system are in chapter 3, "Why Do We Get Sick?"

[4]   Paraphrased from Viktor E. Frankl, *Man's Search for Meaning* (Boston: Beacon Press, 2006).

[5]   Anselm Grün explains this well in *Limites Sanadores/Healing Limits: Estrategias de Autoproteccion/Self-Protection Strategies* (Buenos Aires: Editorial Bonum, 2005).

[6]   Mind-body medicine, as defined by the National Center of Complementary and Alternative Medicine: Practices, uses a variety of techniques to facilitate

the mind's capacity to positively affect bodily functions and symptoms.

[7]   O. Carl Simonton (1942–2009) was an oncologist, author, and lecturer, famous for pioneering studies in psychosocial oncology.

Chapter 5

[1]   *Online Etymology Dictionary.* www.etymonline.com/word/cure

[2]   *Salutogenesis* is a term that was coined by Aaron Antonovsky, physician and sociologist, in the last decades of the twentieth century. See Aaron Antonovsky, *Health, Stress and Coping* (San Francisco: Jossey-Bass, 1979).

[3]   World Health Organization, *Cancer Fact Sheet,* February 2017. www.who.int/mediacentre/factsheets/fs297/en/

[4]   Nearly half the world continues to cook with solid fuels such as dung, wood, agricultural residues, and coal. When used in simple cooking stoves, these fuels release carbon emissions and, on

a global scale, might constitute the largest source of indoor air pollution.

[5]   Dean Ornish et al., "Intensive Lifestyle Changes May Affect the Progression of Prostate Cancer," *Journal of Urology* 174, no.3 (September 2005): 1065–1069; discussion 1069–70. Dean Ornish et al., "Changes in Prostate Gene Expression in Men Undergoing an Intensive Nutrition and Lifestyle Intervention," *Proceedings of the National Academy of Sciences* 105, no.24 (June 17, 2008): 8369–8374. doi:10.1073/pnas.0803080105

[6]   Simone Reuter et al., "Epigenetic Changes Induced by Curcumin and Other Natural Compounds," *Genes & Nutrition* 6, no.2 (May 2011): 93–108. doi:10.1007/s12263-011-0222-1

[7]   Andreas J. Papoutsis et al., "Resveratrol Prevents Epigenetic Silencing of BRCA-1 by the Aromatic Hydrocarbon Receptor in Human Breast Cancer Cells," *Journal of Nutrition* 140, no.9

(September 1, 2010): 1607–1614. doi:10.3945/jn.110.123422

[8] French physician, neuroscientist, and author David Servan-Schreiber was a Professor of Psychiatry and cofounder of the Center for Integrative Medicine at the University of Pittsburgh Medical Center. He was also author of *Healing Without Freud or Prozac: Natural Approaches to Curing Stress, Anxiety and Depression* (London: Pan MacMillan, 2012).

[9] New York: Penguin Books, 2017.

[10] See more about neuronal circuits in chapter 7, "The Treasure Hunt."

[11] American Cancer Society, "Diet and Physical Activity: What's the Cancer Connection?" www.cancer.org/cancer/cancer-causes/diet-physical-activity/diet-and-physical-activity.html

[12] American Cancer Society, "Physical Activity: Cancer Fact Sheet." www.cancer.org/content/dam/cancer-org/cancer-contro

l/en/booklets-flyers/physical-act
ivity-and-cancer-fact-sheet.pdf

[13]   Based on the American Cancer
Society's Guidelines on Nutrition
and Physical Activity for Cancer
Prevention. www.cancer.org/he
althy/eat-healthy-get-active/acs
-guidelines-nutrition-physical-ac
tivity-cancer-prevention.html

[14]   Philip B. Sparling et al.,
"Recommendations for Physical
Activity in Older Adults," *BMJ
(British Medical Journal)* 350:
h100 (January 21, 2015).
Phillipe de Souto Barreto,
"Global Health Agenda on
Non-Communicable Diseases:
Has WHO Set a Smart Goal for
Physical Activity?" *BMJ* 350:
h23 (January 21, 2015).

[15]   Fabiana Benatti and Bente
Klarlund Pedersen, "Exercise as
an Anti-Inflammatory Therapy
for Rheumatic Diseases-Myokine
Regulation," *Nature Reviews
Rheumatology* 11, no.2
(February 2015): 86–97. Julie
Midtgaard et al., "Efficacy of
Multimodal Exercise-Based

Rehabilitation on Physical Activity, Cardiorespiratory Fitness, and Patient-Reported Outcomes in Cancer Survivors: A Randomized, Controlled Trial," *Annals of Oncology* 24, no.9 (September 2013): 2267–2273. Karin M. Thijs et al., "Rehabilitation Using High-Intensity Physical Training and Long-Term Return-to-Work in Cancer Survivors," *Journal of Occupational Rehabilitation* 22, no.2 (June 2012): 20–229. Lis Adamsen et al., "Effect of a Multimodal High Intensity Exercise Intervention in Cancer Patients Undergoing Chemotherapy: Randomised Controlled Trial," *BMJ* 339: b3410 (October 13, 2009).

[16] Ulrica Von Thiele Schwarz and Henna Hasson, "Employee Self-Rated Productivity and Objective Organizational Production Levels: Effects of Worksite Health Interventions Involving Reduced Work Hours and Physical Exercise," *Journal*

of *Occupational and Environmental Medicine* 53, no.8 (August 2011): 838–944. doi:10.1097/JOM.0b013e31822 589c2 and Tim W. Puetz, Sara S. Flowers, and Patrick J. O'Connor, "A Randomized Controlled Trial of the Effect of Aerobic Exercise Training on Feelings of Energy and Fatigue in Sedentary Young Adults with Persistent Fatigue," *Psychotherapy and Psychosomatics* 77, no.3 (2008): 167–174. doi:10.1159/ 000116610

[17] Sterian Elavsky, "Longitudinal Examination of the Exercise and Self-Esteem Model in Middle-Aged Women," *Journal of Sport and Exercise Psychology* 32, no.6 (December 2010): 862–880.

[18] Lynette L Craft and Frank M. Perna, "The Benefits of Exercise for the Clinically Depressed," *Primary Care Companion to the Journal of Clinical Psychiatry* 6, no.3 (2004): 104–111.

[19] A recent meta-analysis on prediabetes and heart diseases found that exercise therapy is as effective as drug therapy. Exercising, by means of myokines, helps normalize insulin, glucose, and leptin levels. This is one of the main effects exercise has to optimize health and prevent chronic diseases, including the metabolic syndrome. Apparently exercising does not reduce leptin levels directly, but through metabolic changes, increase of insulin sensitivity, and improvement of metabolism of fats, among other mechanisms. Huseyin Naci and John P.A. Ioannidis, "Comparative Effectiveness of Exercise and Drug Interventions on Mortality Outcomes: Metaepidemiological Study," *BMJ* 347 (2013): f5577. doi:10.113 6/bmj.f5577 and Robert. R. Kraemer, Hongnan Chu, and V. Daniel Castracane, "Leptin and Exercise," *Experimental Biology*

and Medicine (Maywood) 227, no.9 (October 2002): 701–708.

[20] Karlie A. Intlekofer and Carl W. Cotman, "Exercise Counteracts Declining Hippocampal Function in Aging and Alzheimer's Disease," *Neurobiology of Disease* 57 (September 2013): 47–55. doi:10.1016/j.nbd.2012 .06.011

[21] Seventeenth-century French mathematician, philosopher, and scientist René Descartes influenced Western culture significantly. He laid the basis of Western philosophy; he was the father of analytic geometry and the Cartesian system named after him, and was one of the key representatives of the scientific revolution. His best-known statement, "I think, therefore I am," still influences Western thought.

[22] The basic premises of Newton's laws, also known as Newton's three laws of motion, are that there exists a universal time and that particles follow

well-defined trajectories. They raise the possibility of explaining not only the motion of objects on earth and celestial bodies, but also the operation of machines. Newtonian mechanics help describe everyday phenomena, i.e., those developing at much lower speeds than light and at a macroscopic scale. Newtonian mechanics cannot explain phenomena at a microscopic scale or lower, or at speeds near light, such as the operation of a cell phone. These are explained through Einstein's theory of relativity or quantum physics.

[23] "Who Am I?" written by Emiliano Jimenez Hernández (1941–2007), Spanish priest, missionary, and teacher. He wrote Biblical commentary and theological anthropology, among other subjects. In 2003, after years of missions throughout the world, he returned to Rome, suffering from cancer,

and died four years later. Those who knew him remember his wit, ability to cope with adversity, patience, permanent smile throughout his disease, and his understanding of human frailty.

[24]   In his book *The Web of Life: A New Scientific Understanding of Living Systems* (New York: Anchor Books, 1997), xviii, Fritjof Capra explains: "During the twentieth century, the change from the mechanistic to the ecological paradigm proceeded in different forms.... The basic tension is one between the parts and the whole. The emphasis on the parts has been called mechanistic, reductionist, or atomistic; the emphasis on the whole holistic, organismic, or ecological.... In biology, the tension between mechanism and holism has been a recurring theme throughout its history and is an inevitable consequence of the ancient

dichotomy between substance (matter, structure, quantity) and form (pattern, order, quality)." In *Systems View of Life,* he elegantly describes the systems' view in medicine.

[25]   *Bodywork* or conscious body exercise is a term used to describe any personal or therapeutic development technique involving the body by means of massage, breathing, or energetic therapies. The goal of these techniques is to create awareness of the mind-body or the energetic body. Some of these techniques are Reiki, yoga, pranayama, therapeutic touch, qigong, taiji, bioenergetics, applied physiotherapy, chiropractic, and reflexology.

[26]   See chapter 9, "Tuning Up."

[27]   Peugeot 208 slogan. http://the inspirationroom.com/daily/2011/peugeot-208-let-your-body-drive/

[28]   See, e.g., Alexander Lowen, *Bioenergetics: The*

Revolutionary Therapy That Uses the Language of the Body to Heal the Problems of the Mind (New York: Penguin Books, 1994).

[29]   See more about anti-stress in chapter 9, "Tuning Up."

[30]   Vegetables, and by extension tubers and legumes.

[31]   See "Organic Foods" in the glossary in appendix 1, "Nutrition."

[32]   Cancer Research UK, "Food and Drink to Avoid During Cancer Treatment." www.cancerresearc huk.org/about-cancer/cancer-in -general/treatment/cancer-drug s/how-you-have/taking-medicin es/foods-drinks-avoid

[33]   Adam S. Gardner et al., "Randomized Comparison of Cooked and Noncooked Diets in Patients Undergoing Remission Induction Therapy for Acute Myeloid Leukemia," *Journal of Clinical Oncology* 26, no.35 (December 10, 2008): 5684–5688. doi:10.1200/JCO.2 008.16.4681 and American

Cancer Society, "Infections in People with Cancer," www.canc er.org/treatment/treatments-an d-side-effects/physical-side-effe cts/infections/infections-in-peop le-with-cancer.html

[34] Cancer cells may reschedule the metabolic system to be able to produce energy by glycolysis, even under normal oxygen conditions (Warburg effect). Sugars reduction could block this energy source. Paula Lopez-Serra et al., "A *DERL3*-Associated Defect in the Degradation of SLC2A1 Mediates the Warburg Effect," *Nature Communications* 5, article no.3608 (April 3, 2014). doi:10.1038/ncomms4608

[35] Most people are used to burning sugars or carbohydrates as their main fuel, but they are not used to burning fat. Intermittent fasting is useful to overcome addictions to sweets and to increase the production of enzymes designed to burn fat. One of the most effective

strategies is to limit meals to a six-to-eight-hour period, for example, eating only between 11a.m. and 7p.m. The word *breakfast* means, literally, "to break the fast," to start eating after a night's fast. At first, cutting an addiction to sweets may produce physical discomfort, such as headaches and nausea, typical withdrawal syndromes. Therefore, it is recommended to fast under medical control.

[36] Alina Vrieling et al, "Serum 25-Hydroxyvitamin D and Postmenopausal Breast Cancer Survival: A Prospective Patient Cohort Study," *Breast Cancer Research* 13, no.4 (July 26, 2011): R74. doi:10.1186/bcr2920

[37] Christian Kurts et al., "The Immune System and Kidney Disease: Basic Concepts and Clinical Implications," *Nature Reviews Immunology* 13 (2013): 738–753. doi:10.1038/nri3523

[38] Association of Integrative Oncology, Spain. www.oncologi aintegrativa.org

[39] "Report of a Joint Food and Agricultural Organization/World Health Organization Working Group on Drafting Guidelines for the Evaluation of Probiotics in Food" (London, Ontario, April 30 and May 1, 2002). www.wh o.int/foodsafety/fs_managemen t/en/probiotic_guidelines.pdf

[40] Francesco Russo, Michele Linsalata, and Antonella Orlando, "Probiotics Against Neoplastic Transformation of Gastric Mucosa: Effects on Cell Proliferation and Polyamine Metabolism," *World Journal of Gastroenterology* 20, no.37 (October 7, 2014): 13258–13272. doi:10.3748/wjg .v20.i37.13258. Kan Shida and Koji Nomoto, "Probiotics as Efficient Immunopotentiators: Translational Role in Cancer Prevention," *Indian Journal of Medical Research* 138, no.5 (November 2013): 808–814.

Peter T. *Shyu,* Glenn G. Oyong, and Esperanza C. Cabrera, "Cytotoxicity of Probiotics from Philippine Commercial Dairy Products on Cancer Cells and the Effect on Expression of cfos and cjun Early Apoptotic-Promoting Genes and Interleukin-1 β and Tumor Necrosis Factor-β Proinflammatory Cytokine Genes," *BioMed Research International* 2014 (2014): 491740. doi:10.1155/2014/491740 and Monika Kassayová et al., "Preventive Effects of Probiotic Bacteria Lactobacillus Plantarum and Dietary Fiber in Chemically-Induced Mammary Carcinogenesis," *Anticancer Research* 34, no.9 (September 2014): 4969–4975.

[41] Association of Integrative Oncology, Spain.

[42] Functional foods is a notion originated in Japan to refer to foods specifically developed to promote health and reduce the risk of disease. That's why they

add only biologically active components, such as minerals, vitamins, fatty acids, dietary fiber, antioxidants, and live microorganisms.

[43] Odile Fernández, "Foods to Prevent Cancer," (in Spanish) www.misrecetasanticancer.com/2014/10/10-alimentos-para-el-cancer.html

[44] Odile Fernández's blog is called "My Anticancer Recipes." (See Shopping List in appendix 1, "Nutrition.")

[45] Caroline Davis, "From Passive Overeating to 'Food Addiction': A Spectrum of Compulsion and Severity," *ISRN Obesity* 2013 (2013), article no.435027. doi: 10.1155/2013/435027 and Daniel M. Blumenthal and Mark S. Gold, "Neurobiology of Food Addiction," *Current Opinion in Clinical Nutrition and Metabolic Care* 13, no.4 (July 2010): 359–365. doi:10.1097/MCO.0b013e32833ad4d4

[46]   "Food Additives" (in Spanish). www.aditivos-alimentarios.com/ p/listado-de-aditivos.html

[47]   See "Glutamate and Your Gut: Understanding the Difference Between Umami and MSG," htt ps://bodyecology.com/articles/g lutamate-and-your-gut-understa nding-the-difference-between-u mami-and-msg

[48]   The pH measures the acidity and alkalinity in an aqueous system determined by the number of hydrogen ions. The pH scale spans from 0 to 14: acid substances are those with pH<7 and alkaline those with pH >7; pH=7 is the neutral point. A healthy person has a blood pH value between 7.40 and 7.45, which is slightly alkaline.

[49]   We know that if we increase the cardiac rhythm in excess, we increase the elimination of carbon dioxide, which leads to respiratory alkalosis. The most striking manifestation of respiratory alkalosis is tetany,

a condition marked by intermittent muscular spasms caused by malfunction of the parathyroid glands and a consequent deficiency of ionized calcium.

[50] Foods produce an acidity or alkalinity condition in the organism according to the quality or proteins, carbohydrates, fats, minerals, and vitamins. (See "Alkalize Your Diet" in the glossary in appendix 1.)

[51] Lawrence E, Armstrong et al., "Mild Dehydration Affects Mood in Healthy Young Women," *Journal of Nutrition* 142, no.2 (February 2012): 382–388. doi :10.3945/jn.111.142000

[52] See www.whatthebleep.com

[53] Contemporary Italian physician who was a member of the European Organization for Nuclear Research (CERN) in Geneva, Switzerland.

[54] Adapted from Mae-Wan Ho, *The Rainbow and the Worm: The Physics of Organisms*

(Singapore: World Scientific Publishing Company, 2008).

[55] Adapted from American Cancer Society, "Tobacco and Cancer," www.cancer.org/cancer/cancer-causes/tobacco-and-cancer.html

[56] Mantras are words or phrases that can be repeated aloud or internally as meditations. Through history, different cultures have believed in the sacred power of words and have imagined that by pronouncing certain names or sounds, they could attract different energies, or gods.

[57] Harvard Medical School, "Why Sleep Matters." http://healthysleep.med.harvard.edu/healthy/matters

[58] Laila AlDabal et al., "Metabolic, Endocrine, and Immune Consequences of Sleep Deprivation," *Open Respiratory Medical Journal* 5 (July 23, 2011): 31–43. doi:10.2174/1874306401105010031

[59]   Matthew P. Walker and Els van der Helm, "Overnight Therapy? The Role of Sleep in Emotional Brain Processing," *Psychological Bulletin* 135, no.5 (2009): 731–748. doi:10.1037/a0016570

[60]   See www.dedoublement.com/en

[61]   Sleep deprivation is associated with lower levels of leptin, a hormone that signals to the brain that we're full, and higher levels of ghrelin, the hunger signal.

[62]   WebMD, "Physical Side Effects of Oversleeping," 2012. www.webmd.com/sleep-disorders/guide/physical-side-effects-oversleeping#1

[63]   Dr. Daniel P. Cardinali's blog is an excellent reference for sleep issues. http://daniel-cardinali.blogspot.com.ar*Note:* This web page is in Spanish. For translation, paste the URL in the Google Search block and click "Translate This Page."

[64] L-tryptophan is an essential amino acid. We must add it to our diet. It is necessary in order to produce melatonin and serotonin, hormones involved in the sleep-wakefulness cycle.

[65] Cortisol secretion, which is involved in several biological functions, is programmed for the active period during the day, with a high level of secretion in the morning. Secretion cycles of cortisol and other hormones are regulated precisely, not only by the hypothalamic-pituitary-adrenal axis, but also by the circadian rhythm that depends on exposure to light. Sooyoung Chung, Gi Hoon Son, and Kyungjin Kim, "Circadian Rhythm of Adrenal Glucocorticoid: Its Regulation and Clinical Implications," *Biochimica et Biophysica Acta* 1812, no.5 (May 18, 2011): 581–591. doi:10.1016/j.bbadis. 2011.02.003

[66]   Irina V. Zhdanova et al., "Sleep-Inducing Effects of Low Doses of Melatonin Ingested in the Evening," *Clinical Pharmacology & Therapeutics* 57, no.5 (May 1995): 552–558.

[67]   T. Roth et al., "Benzodiazepines and Memory," *British Journal of Clinical Pharmacology* 18, suppl. 1 (1984): 45S–49S.

[68]   US Food and Drug Administration, "Parabens in Cosmetics." www.fda.gov/cosmetics/productsingredients/ingredients/ucm128042.htm

Chapter 6

[1]   From Naomi Shihab Nye, *Words Under the Words: Selected Poems* (Portland, Oregon: Eighth Mountain Press, 1994). Used with permission of the author.

[2]   It's possible to restore a healthy micro-environment by reducing inflammation, stimulating the immune system, and recovering the circadian rhythms and hormonal cycles.

[3]   See chapter 1, "The Diagnosis Is a Tsunami."

[4]   There is evidence that meditation techniques improve immunological parameters. Linda Ellen Carlson, Michael Speca, Kamala D. Patel, and Eileen Goodey, "Mindfulness-Based Stress Reduction in Relation to Quality of Life, Mood, Symptoms of Stress, and Immune Parameters in Breast and Prostate Cancer Outpatients," *Psychosomatic Medicine* 65, no.4 (July–August 2003): 571–581. Linda E. Carlson, Michael Speca, Peter Faris, and Kamala D. Patel, "One Year Pre–Post Intervention Follow-Up of Psychological, Immune, Endocrine and Blood Pressure Outcomes of Mindfulness-Based Stress Reduction (MBSR) in Breast and Prostate Cancer Outpatients," *Brain, Behavior, and Immunity* 21, no.8 (November 2007): 1038–1049. www.radboudcentru mvoormindfulness.nl/media/Artik

elen/Carlson_Speca_Faris__Patel 2007.pdf

[5]   It has been proven that the immune system induces senescence in tumor cells, thus inhibiting tumor growth without harming healthy cells. Heidi Braumüller, Thomas Wieder, and Martin Röcken, "T-Helper-1-Cell Cytokines Drive Cancer into Senescence," *Nature* 494, no.7437 (February 21, 2013): 361–365. doi:10.1038/nature11824

[6]   See chapter 5, "Energize Your Body!"

[7]   Catherine Classen et al., "Supportive-Expressive Group Therapy and Distress in Patients with Metastatic Breast Cancer: A Randomized Clinical Intervention Trial," *Archives of General Psychiatry* 58, no.5 (May 2001): 494–501.

[8]   Glyphosate, the main component of Roundup herbicide, used widely including for soy cultivation, produces cancer and embryonic abnormalities.

Research studies have been carried out by Andrés Carrasco, a molecular embryologist and neuroscientist who was the head of the Molecular Embryology Lab at University of Buenos Aires (UBA) and chief scientist at the National Council for Science and Technology (Conicet), Argentina. Kathryn Z Guyton et al., "Carcinogenicity of Tetrachlorvinphos, Parathion, Malathion, Diazinon, and Glyphosate," *Lancet Oncology* 16, no.5 (March 20, 2015): 490–491. www.thelancet.com/journals/lanonc/article/PIIS1470-2045(15)70134-8/fulltext

[9]   Many patients are looking for an oncologist to guide them, not only during the process of diagnosis, but also during treatment, someone who will take ongoing care of the patient's active profile and coordinate the specialists involved as results come in. See *El Valor Terapéutico en Oncología (The Therapeutic Value of*

Oncology) (Barcelona: Universidad de los Pacientes, 2009) in Spanish. www.aecc.es/ Nosotros/Nosmovemos/accionesr ealizadas/Documents/2009%20v alor%20terapeutico%20en%20on cologia.pdf

[10] Jeffrey A. Meyerhardt, et al., "Impact of Physical Activity on Cancer Recurrence and Survival in Patients with Stage III Colon Cancer: Findings from CALGB 89803," *Journal of Clinical Oncology* 24, no.22 (August 1, 2006): 3535–3541.

[11] Janushka Naidoo, D.B. Page, and Jedd D. Wolchok, "Immune Modulation for Cancer Therapy," *British Journal of Cancer* 111, no.12 (December 9, 2014): 2214–2219. doi:10.1038/bjc.20 14.348

[12] The Buddha taught the "middle way" of moderation between extremes.

[13] Crystal L. Park, Jennifer Chmielewski, and Thomas O. Blank, "Post-Traumatic Growth: Finding Positive Meaning in

Cancer Survivorship Moderates the Impact of Intrusive Thoughts on Adjustment in Younger Adults," *Psychooncology* 19, no.11 (November 2010): 1139–1147. doi:10.1002/pon.1680

[14]   Thomas Jessy, "Immunity over Inability: The Spontaneous Regression of Cancer," *Journal of Natural Science, Biology and Medicine* 2, no.1 (January–June 2011): 43–49. doi:10.4103/09 76-9668.82318> and see also Kelly A. Turner, *Radical Remission: Surviving Cancer Against All Odds* (San Francisco: Harper One, 2014). Turner, a scientist, compiled many cases of "incurable cancers" that have been cured.

[15]   For an in-depth understanding, see Marilyn Mandala Schlitz, Cassandra Vieten, and Tina Amorok, *Living Deeply: The Art and Science of Transformation in Everyday Life* (Oakland: New Harbinger Publications, 2008).

[16] See Eckhart Tolle, *The Power of Now: A Guide to Spiritual Enlightenment* (Novato, Calif.: New World Library, 2004).

[17] The mucous membrane is the layer of the skin that covers the internal wall of the organs, such as in the mouth or the digestive or respiratory tract.

[18] Cryotherapy has been proven to prevent mucositis, particularly in the administration of 5-fluorouracil chemotherapy.

[19] Although antioxidants (vitamin A, vitamin E, melatonin) at different doses might protect healthy cells and even increase their anticancer effect, there's wide evidence that high-dose antioxidants might interact with radiation's effects on DNA, reducing its effectiveness. Ralph W. Moss, "Should Patients Undergoing Chemotherapy and Radiotherapy Be Prescribed Antioxidants?" *Integrative Cancer Therapies* 5, no.1 (March 1, 2006): 63–82. Ralph W. Moss, "Do Antioxidants

Interfere with Radiation Therapy for Cancer?" *Integrative Cancer Therapies* 6, no.2 (September 1, 2007): 281–292. Isabelle Bairati et al., "Randomized Trial of Antioxidant Vitamins to Prevent Acute Adverse Effects of Radiation Therapy in Head and Neck Cancer Patients," *Journal of Clinical Oncology* 23, no.24 (August 20, 2005): 5805–5813. Oluwadamilola O. Olaku, Mary O. Ojukwu, Farah Z. Zia, and Jeffrey D. White, "The Role of Grape Seed Extract in the Treatment of Chemo/Radiotherapy Induced Toxicity: A Systematic Review of Preclinical Studies," *Nutrition and Cancer* 67 no.5 (April 16, 2015): 730–740.

[20]   www.breastcancer.org/tips/hair_skin_nails/cold-caps

[21]   http://lookgoodfeelbetter.org

[22]   Katherine D. Crew et al., "Randomized, Blinded, Sham-Controlled Trial of Acupuncture for the Management of Aromatase

Inhibitor-Associated Joint Symptoms in Women with Early-Stage Breast Cancer," *Journal of Clinical Oncology* 28, no.7 (March 1, 2010): 1154–1160. doi:10.1200/JCO.2 009.23.4708

Chapter 7

[1]   Deepak Chopra, in the 1989 edition of his book *Quantum Healing: Exploring the Frontiers of Mind/Body Medicine* (New York: Bantam Books, rev. 2015), wrote, "If you think you are only your physical body, which one are you talking about? To the one that existed in 1970, or to the 1987 model? Not even one of the cells existing in your body in 1987 is currently in your body. They have all been replaced."

[2]   *Adapted from* Ervin Laszlo, *Science and the Akashic Field: An Integral Theory of Everything* (Rochester, VT: Inner Traditions, 2007).

[3]   Kirsty L. Spalding et al., "Retrospective Birth Dating of Cells in Humans," *Cell* 122, no.1 (July 15, 2005), 133–143.

[4]   Nassim Haramein, *The Moving Spiraling Solar System* (Greater Awareness TV, 2011). www.yout ube.com/watch?v=znu7UxwAVcc

[5]   Quantum physics studies matter's behavior down to the subatomic scale and up to the cosmic level. It's based on two critical pillars: (1) Particles exchange energy in units called *quanta.* (2) One can't *know* the speed and position of a quantum particle, so descriptions are in terms of probabilities.

[6]   This is known as G-LOC (G-induced loss of consciousness). Acceleration relative to gravity is quantified in G's. One G is equivalent to the pressure applied to the human body by the gravitational constant (9.80665 meters per second2) at sea level, known as "standard gravity." Andrew Tarantola, "Why the Human Body

Can't Handle Heavy Acceleration,"
Gizmodo. https://gizmodo.com/w
hy-the-human-body-cant-handle-
heavy-acceleration-1640491171

[7]   From "Doubling of Time," a
lecture by Jean-Pierre Garnier
Malet in Buenos Aires, March
2015.

[8]   Adapted from Richard Gerber,
*Vibrational Medicine: The #1
Handbook of Subtle-Energy
Therapies* (Rochester, VT: Bear
& Company, 2001) and Amit
Goswami, *The Quantum Doctor:
A Quantum Physicist Explains the
Healing Power of Integral
Medicine* (Newburyport, Mass.:
Hampton Roads Publishing,
2011).

[9]   Growing organisms are shaped
by fields within and around them
that contain the form of the
organism. Morphic fields (from
the Greek *morphe,* form) are
form-shaping fields, patterns, or
order structures that organize
not only living organisms' fields,
but also those of crystals and
molecules. "Each kind of

molecule, each protein, for example, has its own kind of morphic field—hemoglobin field, insulin field, etc.—Likewise, each kind of crystal, each kind of organism, each kind of instinct or pattern of behavior has its own morphic field. So these fields are the organizing fields of nature. There are many kinds of them, because there are many kinds of things and patterns in nature...." From Rupert Sheldrake, *A New Science of Life: The Hypothesis of Morphic Resonance* (Rochester, VT: Park Street Press, 1995). See also Rupert Sheldrake, "Mind, Memory, and Archetype Morphic Resonance and the Collective Unconscious," *Psychological Perspectives* 18, no.1 (Spring 1987): 9–25. www.sheldrake.org /research/morphic-resonance/par t-i-mind-memory-and-archetype- morphic-resonance-and-the-colle ctive-unconscious

[10] This implies that the mind is a spread-out phenomenon

covering all the organism and acts through a complex chemical network formed by information molecules joining all our activities—mental, emotional, and organic.

[11] Neuroscience explains how our brain acts as an adaptive and dynamic synthesizer that allows us to adjust our internal environment according to what's happening in our external environment.

[12] According to Mario Bunge (Argentine philosopher, Professor Emeritus in Philosophy, McGill University, Montreal, Quebec, Canada), the mind, as we are conceiving it currently, is the result of the fusion of several sciences: p s y c h o - n e u r o - immuno-endocrine sociology. www.bcsss.org/dissemination/lectures/vienna-2014-mario-bunge-the-persistence-of-the-mind-body-problem/

[13] *Contact* is a 1997 North American science fiction drama

film, directed by Robert Zemeckis. It's a film adaptation of Carl Sagan's 1985 novel of the same name.

[14] Like a torus, the chakra has a ring or spherical form constantly spinning from inside to outside.

[15] Elizabeth Schermer, *The Chakras and the Human Energy System* (Seattle: Alchemy Mystery School, n.d.). http://th ealchemyschool.com/wp-conten t/uploads/2015/03/Chakra-Han dout.pdf

[16] Inés Olivero, *Qué decimos cuando hablamos. Parecido no es lo mismo* (What we mean when we speak. Similar is not the same.) (Buenos Aires: Gargola, 2011).

[17] From Joseph Campbell, *The Power of Myth* (New York: Anchor Books, 1991). I like to say, "The clue is in those things that make you feel 'wow!' in plenitude."

[18] Adapted from Elizabeth Gilbert, *Eat, Pray, Love: One Woman's*

Search for Everything Across Italy, India and Indonesia (New York: Riverhead Books, 2007).

[19] Lesson 11, from *A Course in Miracles* (Omaha, Neb.: Course in Miracles Society, 2009). Dr. Helen Schucman wrote this book from a process she describes as an inner dictation, from hearing "the Jesus Christ's voice." She refers to herself as a scribe, and she never claimed authorship of the material.

[20] Bruce H. Lipton, *The Biology of Belief: Unleashing the Power of Consciousness, Matter, & Miracles* (Carlsbad, Calif.: Hay House, 2007).

[21] Chopra, *Quantum Healing.*

[22] This ability to change and adjust the nervous system and the PNIE network is known as *neuro-and PNIE-plasticity.*

Chapter 8

[1] Subtitle of *Almagedón,* Spanish-language theatrical production, directed by Daniel

Canney Martorelli. https://elenco todosomosuno.wordpress.com

[2] Interview with Chilean-French film director and spiritual teacher Alejandro Jodorowsky. www.you tube.com/watch?v=URnHaE5fc6k

[3] Keiron Le Grice, *The Rebirth of the Hero: Mythology as a Guide to Spiritual Transformation* (London: Muswell Hill Press, 2013).

[4] (New York: Penguin Classics, 2002), 263.

[5] This subject is explored in Carl Honoré, *In Praise of Slowness: Challenging the Cult of Speed* (San Francisco: HarperOne, 2005). There is also a slow education movement. Slow teaching implies a respect for each child's rhythm and learning times. See Joan Domènech Francesch, *Elogio de la educación lenta (A tribute to slow education)* (Barcelona: Editorial Grao, 2013).

[6] Olivero, *Qué decimos cuando hablamos (What we mean when we speak).*

[7]   Matthew 22:35–40.

Chapter 9

[1]   Goswami, *Quantum Doctor.*
[2]   Thomas   Taylor,   trans.,
        Iamblichus' Life of Pythagoras
        (Rochester, VT: Inner Traditions;
        1986).
[3]   With thanks to Thich Nhat Hanh
        for his many teachings on this.
        See, e.g. *The Miracle of
        Mindfulness* (Boston: Beacon
        Press, 1975).
[4]   Alexander Molassiotis et al., "The
        Effectiveness of Progressive
        Muscle Relaxation Training in
        Managing Chemotherapy-Induced
        Nausea and Vomiting in Chinese
        Breast Cancer Patients: A
        Randomised Controlled Trial,"
        Support Care Cancer 10, no.3
        (April 2002): 237–246. Heather
        Greenlee et al., "Clinical Practice
        Guidelines on the Use of
        Integrative Therapies as
        Supportive Care in Patients
        Treated for Breast Cancer,"
        Journal of the National Cancer

Institute Monographs 2014, no.50 (November 4, 2014).

[5] Linda Carlson et al., "Mindfulness-Based Stress Reduction in Relation to Quality of Life, Mood, Symptoms of Stress, and Immune Parameters in Breast and Prostate Cancer Outpatients," *Psychosomatic Medicine* 65, no.4 (July–August 2003): 571–581.

[6] James E. Stahl, Michelle L. Dossett, A. Scott LaJoie, John W. Denninger, Darshan H. Mehta, Roberta Goldman, Gregory L. Fricchione, and Herbert Benson, "Relaxation Response and Resiliency Training and Its Effect on Healthcare Resource Utilization," *PLOS ONE* 10, no.10 (October 13, 2015).

[7] Irfan Alli, *101 Selected Sayings of Mahatma Gandhi* (eBookIt.com, 2013), 21.

[8] Don Miguel Ruiz, *The Four Agreements: A Practical Guide to Personal Freedom* (San Rafael, Calif.: Amber-Allen Publishing, 1997).

[9]   Breathing exercises centered in the heart can help change attitudes that normally produce stress. See Heartmath Institute (www.heartmath.org), founded in 1991. This institute is devoted to the research and publication of techniques developed to empower people through access to the heart's intuition and intelligence. They refer to the heart's intelligence as the "third brain."

[10]   Peyer's patch (see illus.5 in ch.2, "The PNIE Network") are clusters of lymphoid nodules, similar to tonsils, located along the small intestine.

[11]   The enteric nervous system is a part of the autonomic nervous system covering a large portion of the digestive tract and is in charge of controlling the esophagus, the stomach, the small intestine, and the colon. It is formed by 100 million neurons, the same number as found in the spinal cord.

[12] Daniel Goleman, *Emotional Intelligence: Why It Can Matter More Than IQ* (New York: Bantam Books, 2005).

[13] Goleman, *Emotional Intelligence.*

[14] Daniel Goleman, *Destructive Emotions: A Scientific Dialogue with the Dalai Lama* (New York: Bantam Books, 2004).

[15] Candace B. Pert, *Molecules of Emotion: Why You Feel the Way You Feel* (New York: Pocket Books, 1999).

[16] We already know that chronic stress adversely affects the PNIE network: it depresses the immune system; increases blood pressure, cholesterol levels, and sugar in blood; and produces a hormonal imbalance.

[17] The research of Arvid Carlsson, Paul Greengard, and Eric R. Kandel, recipients of the 2000 Nobel Prize in Physiology "for their discoveries concerning signal transduction in the nervous system," shows how cell receptors store information

based on how many times they've been stimulated, and in this way know if they've been overstimulated. Prior stimulation determines how information flows.

[18]   There is scientific evidence stating that both the prevention and the course of a disease already diagnosed may improve by treating emotion. Nowadays it is unethical not to include treatment for chronic emotional conditions in cardiovascular patients where the emotional impacts are clearly shown. See Goleman, *Emotional Intelligence.*

[19]   Goleman, *Emotional Intelligence.*

[20]   Newton's third law states that for every action, there is an equal and opposite reaction.

[21]   *Interstellar* is a 2014 science fiction film directed, cowritten, and coproduced by Christopher Nolan.

[22]   Carolyn Myss, *Defy Gravity: Healing Beyond the Bounds of*

Reason (Carlsbad, Calif.: Hay House, 2011), 13.

[23] The French phrase *le tu qui tue* literally means "the killing you," suggesting that when we accuse someone, we're killing the relationship.

[24] Marshall B. Rosenberg, *Nonviolent Communication: A Language of Life* (Encinitas, Calif.: Puddledancer Press, 2015).

[25] See www.thetappingsolution.com/what-is-eft-tapping/

[26] Clinical trials have shown that tapping reduces the emotional impact produced by memories or incidents that trigger emotional stress. Dawson Church, Crystal Hawk, Audrey J. Brooks, Olli Toukolehto, Maria Wren, and Phyllis Stein, "Psychological Trauma Symptom Improvement in Veterans Using Emotional Freedom Techniques: A Randomized Controlled Trial," *Journal of Nervous and Mental Disease* 201, no.2 (February 2013): 153–160. https://pdfs.s

emanticscholar.org/da5f/43bcc8
0084453a5a 347eb7296636f26
6a990.pdf

[27]   Flourishing is also known as post-traumatic growth. Tracy J. Connerty and Vikki Knott, "Promoting Positive Change in the Face of Adversity: Experiences of Cancer and Post-Traumatic Growth," *European Journal of Cancer Care* 22, no.3 (May 2013), 334–344. doi:10.1111/ecc.1203 6

[28]   Gregg Braden, *Secrets of the Lost Mode of Prayer: The Hidden Power of Beauty, Blessing, Wisdom, and Hurt* (Carlsbad, Calif.: Hay House, 2016).

[29]   Gaétan Chevalier, Stephen T. Sinatra, James L. Oschman, Karol Sokal, and Pawel Sokal, "Earthing: Health Implications of Reconnecting the Human Body to the Earth's Surface Electrons," *Journal of Environmental and Public Health* 2012, no.291541 (January 12,

2012); doi:10.1155/2012/2915 41 and Epub 2012 Jan 12. doi :10.1155/2012/291541 and James L. Oschman, Gaétan Chevalier, and Richard Brown, "The Effects of Grounding (Earthing) on Inflammation, the Immune Response, Wound Healing, and Prevention and Treatment of Chronic Inflammatory and Autoimmune Diseases," *Journal of Inflammation Research* 24, no.8 (March 2015), 83–96. doi:10.2 147/JIR.S69656

Chapter 10

[1] Miguel de Cervantes Saavedra, trans. John Rutherford, *Don Quixote* (New York: Penguin Classics, 2003); J.R.R. Tolkien, *The Lord of the Rings: 50th Anniversary Edition* (Boston: Houghton Mifflin Harcourt/Mariner Books, 2005); George Lucas, *Star Wars* film series. *Finding Joe,* a film about the life and work of Joseph Campbell by

Patrick Takaya Solomon, explains this clearly.

[2] This practice has been adapted from the SOS course taught by Jean-Pierre Garnier Malet in Madrid, September 2015. See www.desdoblamiento.es/en/workshops-jean-pierre-garnier-malet/sos-workshop

[3] This "butterfly effect" comes from the Chinese proverb, "When a butterfly flaps its wings in one part of the world, it can cause a hurricane in another part of the world." This is a concept of chaos theory, that in certain systems, the smallest change can cause the system to develop in completely different forms. A small change in an initial state, through an amplifying process, can result in a significantly larger effect in the midterm. Thus, it is difficult to predict with certainty the midterm result.

[4] Joan Walsh Anglund.

Appendix 1

[1] See "Antioxidants and Phytochemicals" in the glossary that follows these urban legends.

[2] Elizabeth S. Mitchell, "WATCH: Organic Food Takes on Meaningless 'All Natural' Labels in Snarky Ad," *Adweek* (February 14, 2014). www.adweek.com/dig ital/watch-organic-food-takes-on-meaningless-all-natural-labels-in-snarky-ad/#/

[3] Rainer W. Bussmann, "The Globalization of Traditional Medicine in Northern Peru: From Shamanism to Molecules," in *Evidence-Based Complementary and Alternative Medicine,* 2013 (2013), art. no.291903. http://d x.doi.org/10.1155/2013/291903

[4] See Food Standards Agency, "Current EU Approved Additives and Their E Numbers": www.foo d.gov.uk/science/additives/enum berlist and Codex General Standard for Food Additives, "Food Additives Index": www.fao

.org/gsfaonline/additives/index.h
tml

[5] www.who.int/foodsafety/publicati
ons/jecfa/en/

[6] American Cancer Society, "Food
Additives, Safety, and Organic
Foods." www.cancer.org/healthy/
eat-healthy-get-active/acs-guidel
ines-nutrition-physical-activity-ca
ncer-prevention/food-additives.ht
ml

[7] More information at www.mskcc
.org/cancer-care/integrative-med
icine/herbs/blue-green-algae

[8] There are other types of anemia
that don't depend on the amount
of iron.

[9] N. Nirmal, D. Pugh et al., "Oral
Administration of a Spirulina
Extract Enriched for Braun-Type
Lipoproteins Protects Mice
Against Influenza A (H1N1) Virus
Infection," *Phytomedicine* 22,
no.2 (February 15, 2015):
271–276. doi:10.1016/j.phymed.
2014.12.006

[10] The base or alkalis is the
opposite of acids and refers to

any substance used to alkalize the medium or increase the pH.

[11] Oxidation is a chemical reaction that transfers electrons from a substance to an oxidant. During metabolism, chemical reactions allow for the binding of simpler molecules to form more complex molecules, and for the breaking down of complex molecules into simpler ones. Both simpler and complex molecules need an appropriate number of electrons to remain stable. If a molecule loses one or more electrons, it transforms into a free radical, which will try to combine with other molecules to regain stability. During this search, free radicals may damage other molecules, even DNA, and trigger chain reactions that result in more free radicals.

[12] Plants and animals maintain complex systems of multiple kinds of antioxidants, such as glutathione, vitamin C, and vitamin E, as well as enzymes

such as catalase, superoxide dismutase, and several peroxidases.

[13]   Ralph W. Moss, "Do Antioxidants Interfere with Radiation Therapy for Cancer?" *Integrative Cancer Therapies* 6, no.3 (September 2007): 281–292.

[14]   Erika Loftfield, et al., "Coffee Drinking and Cutaneous Melanoma Risk in the NIH-AARP Diet and Health Study," *Journal of the National Cancer Institute* 107, no.2 (January 20, 2015): doi:10.1093/jnci/dju421

[15]   ACS, "Food Additives."

[16]   Medline Plus, "Dietary Fats Explained." https://medlineplus .gov/ency/patientinstructions/00 0104.htm

[17]   There are many listings of safe and less-safe fish to eat. Here is an example: https://thewhol ejourney.com/finding-healthy-fi sh-avoiding-toxins-mercury-and -radiation/

[18]   See Joseph Mercola, "How to Combine Foods for Optimal

Health," October 27, 2013. htt ps://articles.mercola.com/sites/ articles/archive/2013/10/27/foo d-combining.aspx

[19]   DNA, or deoxyribonucleic acid, is the substance that constitutes our genes and chromosomes, responsible for heredity.

[20]   ACS, "Common Misconceptions."

[21]   Tinctures are liquid extracts made from herbs that you take orally. They're usually extracted in alcohol. Mother tincture refers to a combination of a botanical extract with a specific amount of alcohol.

[22]   Harvard T.H. Chan School of Public Health, "Healthy Eating Plate & Healthy Eating Pyramid." www.hsph.harvard.ed u/nutritionsource/healthy-eating -plate/

[23]   Osteoporosis reduces the tissues that form the bones, the proteins that are their matrix or structure, and the mineral calcium salts contained in it. As the bones become

more fragile, their resistance to falls decreases, and they break more easily.

[24]   *Media* is a term used in science to describe the fluids *around* the cells (not *in* the cells).

[25]   ACS, "Food Additives."

[26]   Centre for Science and Environment (India), "Removing Pesticides from Fruits and Vegetables," www.cseindia.org/node/2681

[27]   See International Agency for Research on Cancer (IARC), Monographs on the Evaluation of Carcinogenic Risks to Humans. http://monographs.iarc.fr/ENG/Monographs/vol112/index.php and Kathryn Z. Guyton et al., "Carcinogenicity of Tetrachlorvinphos, Parathion, Malathion, Diazinon, and Glyphosate," *Lancet Oncology* 16, no.5: 490–491.

[28]   One of my mentors at Memorial Sloan Kettering Cancer Center said this often.

[29]   ACS, "Food Additives."

[30]   ACS, "Food Additives."

[31]   Ketan R Patel et al., "Clinical Pharmacology of Resveratrol and Its Metabolites in Colorectal Cancer Patients," *Cancer Research* 70, no.19 (Oct 1, 2010): 7392–7399. K. Magyar et al., "Cardioprotection by Resveratrol: A Human Clinical Trial in Patients with Stable Coronary Artery Disease," *Clinical Hemorheology and Microcirculation* 50, no.3. (2012): 179–187.

[32]   Richard D. Semba et al., "Resveratrol Levels and All-Cause Mortality in Older Community-Dwelling Adults," *JAMA Internal Medicine* 174, no.7 (2014): 1077–1084. doi:10.1001/jamainternmed.2014.1582

[33]   It was proven in lab research studies that resveratrol has anticancer properties: it inhibits the proliferation of cancer cells through apoptosis (programmed cell death) and anti-estrogenic effects. It may also sensitize those cells resistant to

chemotherapy agents. It was also proven that resveratrol reduces the effectiveness of certain chemotherapies in some tumor cells. See Memorial Sloan Kettering Cancer Center, "Resveratrol." www.mskcc.org/cancer-care/integrative-medicine/herbs/resveratrol

[34] Patrick J. Skerrett, "Resveratrol—the Hype Continues," *Harvard Health* blog (February 3, 2012). www.health.harvard.edu/blog/resveratrol-the-hype-continues-201202034189

[35] *Søren Skov,* "Selenium Compounds Boost Immune System to Fight Against Cancer," University of Copenhagen (November 24, 2014). http://healthsciences.ku.dk/news/news2014/selenium-compounds-boost-immune-system-to-fight-against-cancer/

[36] Michael Hagemann-Jensen et al., "The Selenium Metabolite Methylselenol Regulates the Expression of Ligands That

Trigger Immune Activation through the Lymphocyte Receptor NKG2D," *Journal of Biological Chemistry,* 289 (November 7, 2014), 31576–31590.

[37] National Institutes of Health, "Selenium: Dietary Supplement Fact Sheet." https://ods.od.nih.gov/factsheets/Selenium-HealthProfessional/

[38] Robert H. Lustig, Laura A. Schmidt, and Claire D. Brindis, "Public Health: The Toxic Truth About Sugar," *Nature* 482, no.7383 (February 2, 2012), 27–29. doi:10.1038/482027a

[39] Some diabetic patients have shown an increase of liver, pancreatic, and endometrial cancer, and less frequently, colon, rectal, breast, and bladder cancer. No increase of lung cancer has been detected, and in other cases, e.g., kidney cancer, the correlation is not clear. Edward Giovannucci et al., "Diabetes and Cancer: A Consensus Report," *Diabetes*

Care 33, no.7 (July 2010): 1674–1685. doi:10.2337/dc10-0666

[40] Directly or by means of other growth factors similar to insulin (IGF, insulin-like growth factors).

[41] A recent resurgence of interest in the Warburg hypothesis and cancer metabolism emphasizes the dependence of many cancers on glycolysis for energy, creating a high need for glucose (possibly a "glucose addiction"), since adenosine triphosphate (ATP)-generation by glycolysis requires far more glucose than oxidative phosphorylation, the final metabolic pathway of cellular respiration. Giovannucci et al., "Diabetes and Cancer."

[42] Approved by the US Food and Drug Administration (FDA).

[43] Elena Lecumberri et al., "Green Tea Polyphenol epigallocatechin-3-gallate (EGCG) as Adjuvant in Cancer Therapy," *Clinical Nutrition* 32,

no.6 (December 2013): 894–903. doi:10.1016/j.clnu.2013.03.008

[44] Brahma N. Singh et al., "Black Tea: Phytochemicals, Cancer Chemoprevention, and Clinical Studies," *Critical Reviews in Food Science and Nutrition* 57, no.7 (May 3, 2017): 1394–1410. doi:10.1080/10408398.2014.994700

[45] This has been proven by well-outlined studies. "Curcumin acts against transcription factors, which are like a master switch," said lead researcher Bharat Aggarwal. "Transcription factors regulate all the genes needed for tumors to form. When we turn them off, we shut down some genes that are involved in the growth and invasion of cancer cells." Bharat B. Aggarwal et al., "Curcumin: The Indian Solid Gold," *Advances in Experimental Medicine and Biology* 595 (2007): 1–75.

[46] Joseph Mercola, "Turmeric: The Spice That Actually Doubles as a Powerful Anti-Inflammatory," April 26, 2011. https://articles.mercola.com/sites/articles/archive/2011/04/26/the-spice-that-actually-doubles-as-a-powerful-antiinflammatory.aspx

[47] Memorial Sloan Kettering Cancer Center, "Turmeric." www.mskcc.org/cancer-care/integrative-medicine/herbs/turmeric

[48] American Cancer Society, "Common Misconceptions About Dietary Supplements." www.cancer.org/treatment/treatments-and-side-effects/complementary-and-alternative-medicine/dietary-supplements/misconceptions.html

[49] Attrition rates during tests on substances such as drugs are very high. Ninety-five percent of the molecules tested in Phase 1 anticancer trials do not reach marketing authorization. This makes the drug development process enormously costly and

inefficient. Thomas Hartung. "Food for Thought Look Back in Anger—What Clinical Studies Tell Us About Preclinical Work," *ALTEX: Alternatives to Animal Experimentation* 30, no.3 (October 4, 2013): 275–291. www.altex.ch/resources/raltex_2013_3_275_291_FFTHartung.pdf

[50] See ACS, "Dietary Supplements."

[51] "FDA's Daily Values Fact Sheet." www.accessdata.fda.gov/scripts/InteractiveNutritionFactsLabel/factsheets/Vitamin_and_Mineral_Chart.pdf

[52] Isabelle Bairati et al., "A Randomized Trial of Antioxidant Vitamins to Prevent Second Primary Cancers in Head and Neck Cancer Patients," *JNCI: Journal of the National Cancer Institute* 97, no.7 (April 6, 2005): 481–488. doi:10.1093/jnci/dji095

[53] National Cancer Institute, "Vitamin D and Cancer Prevention." www.cancer.gov/a

bout-cancer/causes-prevention/
risk/diet/vitamin-d-fact-sheet

[54] Eric A Klein et al., "Vitamin E and the Risk of Prostate Cancer: Results of The Selenium and Vitamin E Cancer Prevention Trial (SELECT)," *JAMA: The Journal of the American Medical Association* 306, no.14 (2011): 1549–1556. doi:10.1001/jama.2011.1437

[55] Matthew J. McQueen, Eva Lonn, Hertzel C. Gerstein, Jackie Bosch, and Salim Yusuf, "The HOPE (Heart Outcomes Prevention Evaluation) Study and Its Consequences," *Scandinavian Journal of Clinical and Laboratory Investigation. Supplementum* 240 (2005): 143–56. doi:10.1080/00365510500236366

[56] Katharina Nimptsch, Sabine Rohrmann, and Jakob Linseisen, "Dietary Intake of Vitamin K and Risk of Prostate Cancer in the Heidelberg Cohort of the European Prospective Investigation into Cancer and

Nutrition (EPIC-Heidelberg)," *American Journal of Clinical Nutrition* 87, no.4 (April 2008): 985–992.

[57] American Cancer Society, *Guidelines on Nutrition and Physical Activity for Cancer Prevention: Reducing the Risk of Cancer with Healthy Food Choices and Physical Activity.* www.cancer.org/content/dam/cancer-org/cancer-control/en/presentations/nutrition-and-physical-activity-presentation.pdf

[58] National Institutes of Health, "Zinc: Fact Sheet for Consumers." https://ods.od.nih.gov/factsheets/Zinc-Consumer/

Appendix 2

[1] Hagemann-Jensen et al., "Selenium Metabolite..." (see n.36 in appendix 1). Studies on patients suffering from lymphoma who have received chemo show that selenium enhanced the response to treatment. (Inas A. *Asfour* et al., "High-Dose Sodium

Selenite Can Induce Apoptosis of Lymphoma Cells in Adult Patients with Non-Hodgkin's Lymphoma," *Biological Trace Element Research* 127, no.3 (March 2009): 200–210. doi:10.1007/s1 2011-008-8240-6 and Inas A. Asfour et al., "The Impact of High-Dose Sodium Selenite Therapy on bcl-2 Expression in Adult Non-Hodgkin's Lymphoma Patients: Correlation with Response and Survival," *Biological Trace Element Research* 120 (1–3) (2007): 1–10.) A recent study, however, showed that selenium and vitamin E do not reduce the risk of prostate cancer: Scott M. Lippman et al., "Effect of Selenium and Vitamin E on Risk of Prostate Cancer and Other Cancers: The Selenium and Vitamin E Cancer Prevention Trial (SELECT)," *JAMA: Journal of the American Medical Association* 301, no.1 (January 7, 2009): 39–51. doi:10.1001/jama.2008.8 64

[2]   Demetrius Albanes et al., "Alpha-Tocopherol and Beta-Carotene Supplements and Lung Cancer Incidence in the Alpha-Tocopherol, Beta-Carotene Cancer Prevention Study: Effects of Base-Line Characteristics and Study Compliance," *Journal of the National Cancer Institute* 88, no.21 (November 6, 1996): 1560–1570.

[3]   Isabelle Bairati et al., "Randomized Trial of Antioxidant Vitamins to Prevent Acute Adverse Effects of Radiation Therapy in Head and Neck Cancer Patients," *Journal of Clinical Oncology* 23, no.24 (August 20, 2005): 5805–5813.

[4]   A clinical trial showed that homeopathy may help for dermatitis (skin inflammation) during radiation therapy. Augusta Balzarini et al., "Efficacy of Homeopathic Treatment of Skin Reactions During Radiotherapy for Breast Cancer: A Randomised, Double-Blind Clinical Trial," *British Homeopathic*

Journal 89, no.1 (January 2000): 8–12.) Another research study showed that a homeopathic complex, Cocculine, is not effective in the treatment of nausea and vomiting induced by chemotherapy (David Pérol et al., "Can Treatment with Cocculine Improve the Control of Chemotherapy-Induced Emesis in Early Breast Cancer Patients? A Randomized, Multi-Centered, Double-Blind, Placebo-Controlled Phase III Trial," *BMC Cancer* 12, no.1 (December 17, 2012): 603. There are preliminary studies postulating that homeopathy may improve fatigue and life quality in cancer patients, but this has not been investigated in randomized clinical studies (Matthias Rostock et al., "Classical Homeopathy in the Treatment of Cancer Patients—A Prospective Observational Study of Two Independent Cohorts," *BMC Cancer* 11 (January 17, 2011): 19.

[5] The shiitake mushroom and its active compound, lentinan, have been studied thoroughly in the lab and have been shown to have anticancer properties. Mah-Lee Ng and Ann-Teck Yap, "Inhibition of Human Colon Carcinoma Development by Lentinan from Shiitake Mushrooms (Lentinus edodes)," *Journal of Alternative and Complementary Medicine* 8, no.5 (October 2002): 581–589. T. Okamoto et al., "Lentinan from Shiitake Mushroom (Lentinus edodes) Suppresses Expression of Cytochrome P450 1A Subfamily in the Mouse Liver," *BioFactors* 21, nos.1–4 (2004): 407–409.

[6] Lentinan is a polysaccharide deriving from shiitake that could be responsible for its beneficial effects, including improvements of quality of life and life expectancy of patients with the following types of cancer:

Liver—Noto Isoda et al., "Clinical Efficacy of Superfine Dispersed

Lentinan (beta-1, 3-glucan) in Patients with Hepatocellular Carcinoma," *Hepato-Gastroenterology* 56, no.90 (March–April 2009): 437–441. *Gastric*—Koji Oba et al., "Individual Patient Based Meta-Analysis of Lentinan for Unresectable/Recurrent Gastric Cancer," *Anticancer Research* 29, no.7 (July 29, 2009): 2739–2745. *Colorectal*—Shoichi Hazama et al., "Efficacy of Orally Administered Superfine Dispersed Lentinan (beta-1, 3-glucan) for the Treatment of Advanced Colorectal Cancer," *Anticancer Research* 29, no.7 (July 2009): 2611–2617. *Pancreatic*—Kyoko Shimizu et al., "Efficacy of Oral Administered Superfine Dispersed Lentinan for Advanced Pancreatic Cancer," *Hepato-Gastroenterology* 56, no.89 (January–February, 2009): 240–244.

[7]   A shiitake extract reduced the incidence of adverse effects in patients with advanced gastrointestinal cancer undergoing chemotherapy. Kiyotaka Okuno and K. Uno,

"Efficacy of Orally Administered Lentinula Edodes Mycelia Extract for Advanced Gastrointestinal Cancer Patients Undergoing Cancer Chemotherapy: A Pilot Study," *Asian Pacific Journal of Cancer Prevention* 12, no.7 (2011): 1671–1674.

[8] It's been shown that maitake D fraction stimulates the immune system in animals. An uncontrolled brief study observed that maitake extract could improve symptoms and even produce tumor regression. (Noriko Kodama, Kiyoshi Komuta, and Hiroaki Nanba, "Can Maitake MD-Fraction Aid Cancer Patients?" *Alternative Medicine Review* 7, no.3 (June 1, 2002): 236–239. https://pdfs.semantics cholar.org/5796/b53fa21d843a4f a0084ed99b031a817fc773.pdf. Another study in post-menopausal women with breast cancer observed that the administration of maitake extract showed immunomodulatory effects. Gary E. Deng et al., "A

Phase I/II Trial of a Polysaccharide Extract from Grifola Frondosa (Maitake Mushroom) in Breast Cancer Patients: Immunological Effects," *Journal of Cancer Research and Clinical Oncology* 135, no.9 (September 2009): 1215–1221. Even though some effects on the immune system in humans have been observed, no serious studies have yet shown its application in cancer prevention or treatment. Some studies are being conducted in this respect. More references at www.cancer.org

[9] In Asia, maitake mushroom is used to treat hypertension and diabetes. Maitake may not be adequate for persons taking hypoglycemic medications, since they have synergic effects. S. Konno et al., "A Possible Hypoglycaemic Effect of Maitake Mushroom on Type 2 Diabetic Patients," *Diabetic Medicine* 18, no.12 (December 2001): 1010. Maitake might interfere with

warfarin, increasing the INR (M.R. Hanselin et al., "INR Elevation with Maitake Extract in Combination with Warfarin," *Annals of Pharmacotherapy* 44, no.1 (January 2010): 223–224.

[10]   See Memorial Sloan Kettering Cancer Center, "Graviola," www.mskcc.org/cancer-care/integrative-medicine/herbs/graviola

[11]   Hartung, "Food for Thought."

[12]   When a person is under treatment with Viscum, medications deriving from cytochrome P450 3A4 must be taken with care, since Viscum may increase the secondary effects of these medications.

Appendix 3

[1]   The descriptions of the chakras in this appendix are based on Lucas Cervetti, *Amor, La Luz de la Conciencia (Love, the Light of Awareness),* available for audio download on amazon.com. I recommend his music, "Healing Frequencies," to nourish and

balance the chakras, posted on www.youtube.com/watch?v=kHj9 NcIVzlo Lucas Cervetti's website is www.lucascervetti.com

ABOUT THE AUTHOR

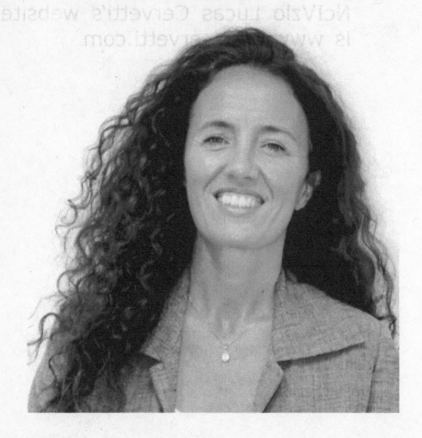

M. LAURA NASI, MD, is an integrative oncologist in private practice in Buenos Aires, Argentina. She specialized in Internal Medicine at Temple University in Philadelphia and in Clinical Oncology at the Memorial Sloan Kettering Cancer Center in New York, was Clinical Research Coordinator for the International Breast Cancer Study Group in Bern, and Research

Director for a Swiss pharmaceutical company. Laura raised two "daughters of the heart" and now lives with her partner, Fernando, alongside a lake on the outskirts of Buenos Aires, where she grows her own vegetables.

About North Atlantic Books

North Atlantic Books (NAB) is an independent, nonprofit publisher committed to a bold exploration of the relationships between mind, body, spirit, and nature. Founded in 1974, NAB aims to nurture a holistic view of the arts, sciences, humanities, and healing. To make a donation or to learn more about our books, authors, events, and newsletter, please visit www.northatlan ticbooks.com.

***

North Atlantic Books is the publishing arm of the Society for the Study of Native Arts and Sciences, a 501(c)(3) nonprofit educational organization that promotes cross-cultural perspectives linking scientific, social, and artistic fields. To learn how you can support us, please visit our website.

BACK COVER MATERIAL

"Dr. Laura Nasi is an internationally recognized figure in the field of integrative medicine. Her book is intended for patients and family members dealing with cancer and is a must-read for medical oncologists and health professionals. It is a welcome addition to the library of anyone interested in a holistic approach to cancer care or just simply interested in living a better and healthier life."

—Gary K. Schwartz, MD, Chief of Hematology and Oncology, Columbia University School of Medicine, New York

AN ONCOLOGIST'S INTEGRATIVE APPROACH TO TREATING AND LIVING *BETTER* WITH OR BEYOND CANCER

In *Cancer as a Wake-Up Call*, Dr. M. Laura Nasi presents a new way of looking at how we view and treat cancer. With current advances in medicine, we're learning more about the ways different aspects of our lives and health impact and interact with one another—why does one long-term smoker get diagnosed with stage-4 lung cancer while another remains cancer-free? Why does someone exposed to a known carcinogen get sick while someone else is apparently immune? What seemingly unrelated factors end up playing key roles in disease etiology, progression, and prognosis?

In this well-researched, inspiring, and easy-to-read guide, Dr. Nasi offers an integrative, whole-person approach to cancer and explains how it is a systemic disease manifesting a global condition locally. Conventional medicine focuses on attacking malignant cells. Integrative medicine encourages chemo and radiation when necessary, while also focusing on a patient's internal balance to help halt the disease. Nasi draws on the latest research on the PNIE (psychoneuro-immuno-endocrine) network to help our systems recognize, repair, or eliminate the cancer cells, focusing on nutrition, stress management, exercise, adequate sleep, healthy relationships, and other body/mind/spirit modalities. Dr. Nasi encourages patients to become empowered agents of their own care.

body/mind/spirit modalities, Dr. Nasi encourages patients to become empowered agents of their own care.

CPSIA information can be obtained
at www.ICGtesting.com
Printed in the USA
BVHW071050121022
649147BV00028B/1525